Naked: Botanical Recipes for Vibrant Skin and Healthy Hair
Copyright © 2015 Elaine Sheff

All photographs by the author except as follows:
Winding path with white flowers: © stenic56, Essential oil bottle with herbs: © Melissa Raimondi | Dreamstime.com, Flour in wooden bowl: © Daizuoxin | Dreamstime.com, Coconut oil: © Geografika | Dreamstime.com, Avocado: © Cwastudios | Dreamstime.com, Almonds: © Karuppasamy .g | Dreamstime.com., Eucalyptus leaves and oil: © PhotoSGH, Elaine Sheff, Arnica: © John Goicovich

Book designed by Elaine Sheff

All rights reserved. No part of this book may be reproduced by any mechanical, photographic or electronic process, or in the form of a recording nor may it be otherwise copied for public or private use, without the prior written permission of the author other than for fair use as brief quotations in articles and reviews.

Naked: Botanical Recipes for Vibrant Skin and Healthy Hair is for educational purposes only. The author does not intend this information to diagnose, cure or prevent any disease or as a substitute for advice provided by your doctor or other health care professional. If you have or may have a serious health care issue, contact your health care provider. Remember to consult with a health care professional before using any natural remedy especially if you are pregnant, nursing or have a serious health concern. If a condition persists, please contact your physician or health care provider. The information provided in this book is not a substitute for a face-to-face consultation with a health care provider, and should not be construed as individual medical advice. Green Path Herb School, Inc., their owners and employees shall not be liable for damage, injury or loss allegedly arising from the information contained in *Naked: Botanical Recipes for Vibrant Skin and Healthy Hair*.

Published by Green Path Herb School, Inc. GreenPathHerbSchool.com
PO Box 7813, Missoula, MT 59807

ISBN: 978-0692342022

This book is dedicated to my sons, Gavin and Zane.
They are my greatest loves and my most profound teachers. They inspire me to continue to make the world a better place in all the small ways I can.
They give me laughter, lightness, and optimism.
I strive to contribute to a hope-filled future for them and their generation.

To all women everywhere, no matter your culture, skin color, age or body type. No matter what television, the media or society may say,
may you know that you are deeply beautiful, inside and out.

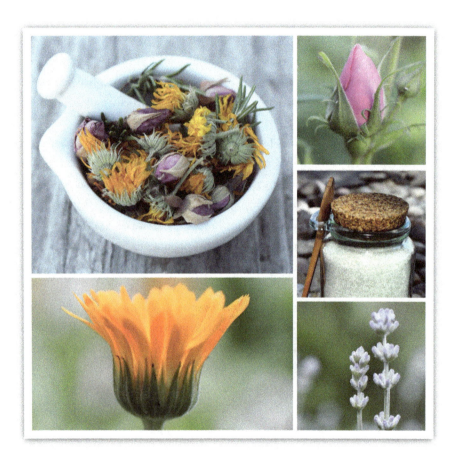

Acknowledgements

I would like to thank the following people for their help and support in writing this book. For many edits, John Goicovich, Christine Sheff, Lynn Purl, Elisabeth Sheff, Nicole Barlow, and Sadie Taylor. For inspiring me on the road to writing my own books and being such an amazing mentor, Rebecca Holman. For my many herb students for trying so many of my recipes with me, and having fun in the kitchen. For Brigitte Mars and Jeanne Rose for being so kind and generous to write reviews for my book. For Karrie Westwood for her cleansing ritual, for taking up the gauntlet and freeing up my time and having the best herbs, essential oils and body care supplies in town.

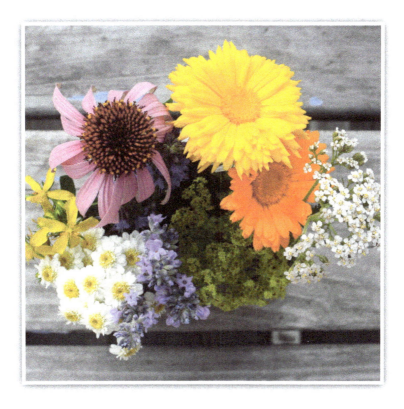

Contents

ACKNOWLEDGEMENTS	3
CONTENTS	4
INTRODUCTION	7
SKIN HEALTH	8
TOOLS	10
HELPFUL MEASUREMENTS	15
CLEANUP STRATEGIES	16
INGREDIENTS	17
SKIN IRRITANTS AND ALLERGENS	18
HERBS	19
CLAYS	29
NATURAL COLORANTS	32
ESSENTIAL OILS	36
NATURAL SALTS	41
FIXED OILS	44
BUTTERS	48
TEMPERING BUTTERS:	48
NATURAL THICKENERS	52
OTHER NATURAL PRODUCTS FOR THE SKIN	55
NATURAL PRESERVATIVES	60
PRESERVATION SUGGESTIONS	63
SKIN TYPES	64
NORMAL SKIN	65
OILY OR PROBLEM SKIN	66
DRY OR SENSITIVE SKIN	68
MATURE SKIN	70
RECIPES FOR THE BODY	71
HERBAL OILS	72
ALOE VERA GEL	76
HEALING GARDEN SALVE	78
DEEP MUSCLE SALVE	80
GREEN BIOTIC OINTMENT	82
AROMATIC CHEST RUB	84
MOISTURIZING LOTION BAR	86
LOTION BAR VARIATIONS:	88
Sunscreen or Diaper Rash Bar	88

  Exfoliating Bar 88
  Bug Repellant Bar 88
  Deodorant Bar..*88*
 SHEA LAVENDER WHIPPED BODY BUTTER 90
 TROPICAL BODY BUTTER..93
 ECZEMA BALM...95
 SOOTHING SITZ BATH..97
 VARICOSE VEIN REFRESHER..100
 CITRUS ALMOND BODY SCRUB 102
  Citrus Body Oil *104*
 SUGAR AND SPICE BODY SCRUB 105
 SPARKLE BODY POWDER 107
 BUG BE GONE OIL..109

RECIPES FOR THE FACE 111
 ALMOND CREAM CLEANSER..112
 VITAMIN C SERUM..114
 LAVENDER FACE TONER 117
 NOURISHING LOTION...119
 BLEMISH BUSTER BALM..122
 BEAT THE HEAT SPRAY..124
 GENTLE EXFOLIATING GRAINS 126
 FRUITY FACEMASK...128
 MINTY TOOTH POWDER...130
 MY FAVORITE LIP BALM RECIPE 132
 LOVELY LIPS BALM...134

RECIPES FOR THE BATH...136
 BLISSFUL BATH 137
 STRESS RELIEF BATH...139
 ROSE CREAM BATH 141
 FOREST GROVE BATH MELTS 143
 SLEEPY BABY BATH 145
 DETOX VINEGAR BATH...147
 HERBAL BATH BOMBS...149
 SORE FOOT SOAK..152
  Sinus Steam *153*
 ACHE NO MORE BATH..154
 SCENTUAL BATH...156
 WAKE ME UP BATH...158
  Wake Me Up Scrub...*159*

RECIPES FOR THE HAIR...160
 HORSETAIL HAIR RINSE 161

- Natural Lice Treatments 163
  - Lice Spray 165
  - Lice Rinse 165
  - Lice Oil *165*
- Healthy Hair Oil 166
- Healthy Hair Oil Variations: 167
  - Dandruff or Fungal Infection of the Scalp 167
  - Hair Growth 167
  - Dark Hair 167
  - Light Hair *168*
- No More Flakes 169

IN CLOSING 172
A BLESSING FOR THE BODY 173
INDEX 174
RECOMMENDED RESOURCES 185
LEARN MORE ABOUT HERBS 188
ABOUT THE AUTHOR 189

Introduction

The skin is the largest organ of the body. It is also one of our main digestive and eliminatory organs. Our first line of defense, the skin protects us from everything from dehydration to overheating as well as bacteria, viruses, fungi and other foreign invaders.

I think of our skin as an outer reflection of our internal health. The condition of the skin can help us know how well our bodies are functioning and eliminating wastes. When working on health care issues, it can be extremely beneficial to include external treatments when applicable. Working both internally and externally on our health often speeds the healing process.

Working both internally and externally on our health often speeds the healing process.

Many products that we put on our skin can be absorbed directly into our bodies and some body care products claiming to be "natural" actually contain harsh chemicals. This is why it is very important to get educated about skin care ingredients and think carefully about what we use on our skin. Often, simple, basic recipes made with ingredients we can pronounce are the best.

The recipes in this book will keep your skin looking and feeling its best, without compromising your health or the health of our beautiful planet. So have fun, get creative, and enjoy the simplicity of making your own safe, effective, inexpensive body care products.

Skin Health

The skin is a living organ that is always changing and adapting to our internal and external environments. For this reason, the skin goes through its own cycles and adjustments. Normal skin cells mature and replace dead skin every 28–30 days.

The skin has several jobs, or functions, in the body. As an immune organ, it is the body's first line of defense against microorganisms, water loss and environmental factors such as harsh weather and pollution. It is one of our major eliminatory organs, producing sweat and releasing waste products. When we need to release especially large amounts of waste products, we may end up with rashes, hives, or skin blemishes. The skin helps maintain homeostasis in the body such as by helping with temperature control by sweating or shivering.

We can even think of the skin as a digestive organ. It is crucial for vitamin D production (try to get moderate sun exposure of about 20 minutes a day) and oxygen absorption. The skin is permeable and can take in chemicals, preservatives, synthetic colorants, petroleum, alcohols, xenoestrogens, and synthetic fragrances. Think about what you want in your body when you put things on your skin!

Healthy skin really comes from the inside of the body. Some of the best things you can do for skin health are to drink plenty of water, get enough sleep, have a bowel movement every day and eat mostly whole, healthy foods, with a focus on fresh vegetables and fruits and good quality oils. Important nutrients to eat for good skin health include protein, B vitamins, vitamins C, D3, E, and K, and essential fatty acids.

Encouraging elimination and sweating (baths are great for this) are important to maintain skin health. Stimulating circulation to the skin with exercise and dry brushing are helpful for vibrant skin. When dry brushing, use a soft, natural bristle brush. Stand naked and move the brush gently from your extremities, starting at your hands and feet, in toward your heart. This will help move the lymph and enhance circulation to the skin.

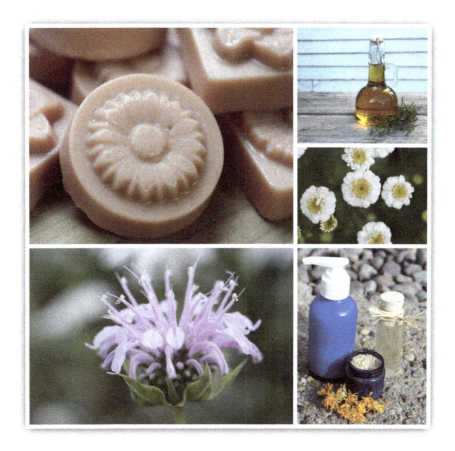

Tools

These tools will make it easier for you to mix and create your own body care products. Many of them may already be in your kitchen.

Coffee grinder, blender, or food processor
These are useful tools for grinding natural ingredients such as salt and herbs or blending a lotion. Although a little harder to use, a mortar and pestle is another useful tool for grinding herbs. Some people prefer dedicated tools for making body care products so as not to impart flavors or odors into foods.

Sharp knife
This tool is essential for cutting herbs and other ingredients such as butters into smaller pieces.

Flat-head screwdriver and hammer
I like to use a flat-head screwdriver and a hammer to break beeswax into smaller chunks. Some people prefer cheese graters for beeswax but I find them tedious and I have grated more than one knuckle trying to use one. If you melt your beeswax in a double boiler before adding your additional ingredients, it is unnecessary to grate it.

Whisk or large spoon
I like stainless steel kitchen tools for mixing ingredients. Although not necessary, a whisk can be very useful at times. It can help to mix powders well, or help add air to lotions and butters. Avoid wood or plastic utensils as they can harbor bacteria and absorb some fixed and essential oils.

Large bowl
Useful for mixing ingredients, I recommend using glass or stainless steel and avoiding aluminum and plastic, as they are more reactive to some fixed and essential oils.

Measuring cups
My favorite type of measuring cups for any kind of herbal medicine making are glass. I especially like Pyrex measuring cups as they can withstand relatively high temperatures.

Measuring spoons
Again, I recommend stainless steel and would avoid plastic, especially for measuring essential oils.

Scoops
Scoops can be useful both for measuring out ingredients and for dispensing the finished product. I have a large stainless steel scoop I use for dry ingredients. I especially like wooden or bamboo scoops for dispensing recipes such as bath salts, face grains, and body scrubs.

Glass jars with tight-fitting lids
This setup is especially important for products with essential oils in them. There are many beautiful containers available. I like small, wide mouth canning jars with plastic lids, which are less reactive than metal lids for long-term storage. If you know someone with a small child, baby food jars work great too. Remember to be careful with glass around the bathtub.

Labels
Always label and date all herbal products that you make. Be sure to include the date and all ingredients on your labels as well. I can't tell you how many times I have made something and thought I would remember the details of my herbal product only to come back to it later and wish I had written it down.

Molds
Useful for body bars, bath melts, and bath bombs, molds can be fashioned from a variety of things. Some of my favorites include molds for candy or glycerin soap and tins for mini muffins. For bath bombs small paper cups work well, as do plastic Easter eggs, which can be held upright in an egg

carton while drying. With hot ingredients, stay away from thin molds that could melt.

Notebook
I encourage you to write down your recipes! It is helpful to have a dedicated notebook for all of your herbal creations. I like to write notes after the recipe describing how it turned out, how I liked it, what the shelf life was and how or if I might change it in the future.

Candy thermometer
Helpful for measuring the temperature of hot oil and other liquids, candy thermometers are also useful for making herbal cough drops.

Double boiler
A saucepan with a detachable upper compartment, double boilers are an ideal way to heat oils, waxes and butters without getting them too hot. The lower pan is partially filled with water and brought to a boil. The upper pan holds the ingredients to be melted. Make sure the pan is stainless steel. It is important to wipe the bottom of the upper pan with a cloth before pouring so as not to get water from the pan bottom in your recipe.

Strainer
Strainers are helpful for straining herbs from teas or oils. I recommend getting a larger stainless steel strainer that is at least eight inches in diameter. Make sure that the strainer is made of fine mesh so that it will catch small pieces of herb or particulate.

Funnel
A small funnel can be helpful for putting both dry and wet recipes into small jars and bottles. If you will be working with essential oils, I would recommend stainless steel or brass over plastic.

Glass dropper
A glass dropper can be very useful for measuring out drops of essential oils or

getting recipes into small bottles. Droppers can be taken apart and cleaned easily for reuse. Be cautioned that essential oils will eventually degrade the rubber tops of droppers.

Muslin or cheesecloth

Useful for straining oils and teas, muslin cloth can also be used in an herb press. I like to line a strainer with muslin before straining oils. Muslin makes an inexpensive bath sachet. It is helpful to use muslin or cheesecloth to cover a fresh plant oil when steeping. Make sure to purchase unbleached material that has not been dyed, as you do not want dyes to leach into your body care products. Wash the material well first, as conventional cotton is grown with lots of pesticides. Get organic material if you can.

Coffee filters

I like unbleached, basket coffee filters for filtering out teas, herbal oils or other sediment. You can set a filter in a strainer or large funnel and let it drain into a bowl or jar. Be warned that this can take some time, so patience is needed.

Digital kitchen scale

Although you can use another type of scale in a pinch, if you are going to make your own body care products or other herbal products with any regularity, I recommend a digital kitchen scale with several important features. It is best if it measures in both ounces and grams and is accurate to the nearest gram and $1/10^{th}$ of an ounce. I like scales that use an electric power cord, but having an option of batteries is nice, too. I recommend a scale that weighs up to at least 1 pound or 454 grams. A tare feature, which allows you to subtract the container weight, is useful. Make sure the platform of the scale is large enough to hold your materials when weighed; I like at least 6 inches square.

pH strips

pH strips are pieces of paper that change color depending on the acidity or alkalinity of a liquid. They can be useful to test some body care products to make sure their pH is within proper limits for stability or effectiveness of the product. Make sure you get strips for the specific range of pH you are looking for, such as from 2.8–4.4 for the vitamin C serum. pH strips can be found at some pharmacies, homebrew stores or online.

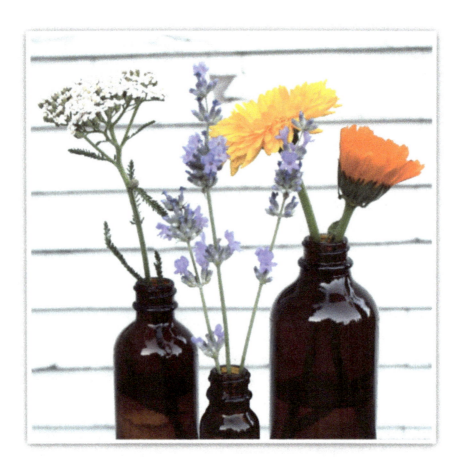

Helpful Measurements

It is useful to have a few basic measurement conversions when making your own natural body care products. These are the measurements I use most frequently. Some ingredients will usually be measured by weight, such as herbs, butters, and beeswax. These ingredients will need to be weighed on a scale. Other ingredients are generally measured by volume including most oils and other liquids. These ingredients will be measured using measuring cups, measuring spoons and droppers. Interestingly, I have found the weights of most oils and butters to be approximately the same as their volumes.

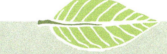

Common Measurements

Weight:
- 16 ounces = 1 pound, 454 grams
- 1 ounce = 28.35 grams

Volume:
- 1 liter = 4.23 cups
- 1 quart = 4 cups, 32 ounces, 0.946 liter
- 1 pint = 2 cups, 16 ounces, 0.473 liter
- 1 cup = 8 ounces, ½ pint, 225 ml
- ½ cup = 4 ounces, 8 tablespoons, 118 ml
- 1 ounce = 2 tablespoons, 29.6 ml
- 1 tablespoon = 3 teaspoons, ½ ounce, 15 ml, about 300 drops
- 1 teaspoon = 5 ml, about 100 drops
- 1 ml = 20-40 drops, depending on the viscosity of the liquid. Thicker liquids yield larger drops.

CLEANUP STRATEGIES

Cleaning up after oils, butters, and beeswax can be a tedious process. As I have done it quite a bit of this over the years, I thought I'd share my best practices with you! I like to use environmentally friendly, low impact, simple cleaners that work well.

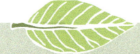

BEST PRACTICES FOR CLEANING UP

Tools:

- Unbleached paper towels (the unbleached part is simply my preference as it helps to reduce toxic chemicals in our environment).
- Baking soda
- Vinegar
- Citrus based natural cleaner and degreaser
- Rubbing alcohol
- Dish soap
- Sponge
- Hot water

How to Use Them:

1. Wipe all oily containers and pans out with paper towels. This significantly reduces your clean up time and water usage.
2. Add some baking soda and vinegar and scrub well with a sponge.
3. Rinse with hot water. This is the first time you will introduce water in the process, as oil and water don't mix well.
4. Pour a little citrus cleaner and dish soap into each container and wash well.
5. Rinse with hot water.
6. For very small containers such as essential oil bottles, start with pouring a little rubbing alcohol into each bottle, shake and drain. Then follow the above process.

Ingredients

Choose your ingredients with care, as these formulas will only be as high quality as the ingredients you use to make them. I have some general recommendations to help you with this process.

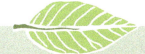

Ingredient Recommendations

- Make sure all your ingredients are fresh.
- Use fresh, cold-pressed vegetable oils that have not been exposed to heat or intense pressure.
- Purchase high quality, pure essential oils. Oils purchased from a trusted source that have been tested using gas chromatography are best.
- Use freshly dried, organic herbs. To maintain freshness, it is better to purchase herbs in a more whole form and grind them yourself when possible.
- Use organic ingredients whenever possible.
- It is best to store these recipes in dark glass containers to protect them from evaporation and light degradation.
- Choose containers that just hold your ingredients and recipes, leaving little space for extra air, which encourages degradation more quickly.
- Make sure ingredients and recipes are kept cool and not exposed to light. Store them in a dark bin, cabinet or in the refrigerator. Some ingredients such as herbs can also be stored in the freezer.

Skin Irritants and Allergens

Some skin care products contain additives that can cause irritation or allergic reactions. If a product is causing redness, itching, scaliness, rash, hives or blisters, discontinue use immediately. Although reactions can be different for each person, the list of common skin irritants includes synthetic fragrances, artificial colorants and dyes, preservatives, parabens, alcohol, formaldehyde releasers, and acids.

According to the American Academy of Dermatology, fragrances cause more allergic contact dermatitis than any other ingredient. If you are sensitive to smells, you may want to reduce the amount of the essential oils suggested in the recipes in this book, or leave them out altogether.

If you have sensitive skin, test your product first by applying a small amount to your inner elbow and waiting 24 hours. If you see redness or irritation, avoid the product and note the ingredients. This can help you narrow down which ingredient is causing a reaction.

If you are allergic or sensitive to a food, I recommend you eschew body care products containing that ingredient. Not because most foods can go through the skin, but because we often touch our mouths or our food with our hands. It is too easy to ingest an allergen if you have it on your person. Interestingly, all of the ingredients listed in this book, as well as all of the recipes are gluten free. The simple nature of the recipes in this book makes it easy to make substitutions and avoid allergens.

There are a few skin care ingredients that are best avoided by everyone. Some of the ingredients to avoid in body care products include synthetic fragrances, sodium lauryl sulfate, sodium laureth sulfate, petrochemicals, polyethylene glycol, lead, propylene glycol, FD & C color pigments, DEA (diethanolamine), MEA (monoethanolamine), TEA (triethanolamine), imidazolidinyl urea, DMDM hydantoin, isopropyl alcohol, formaldehyde, phthalates and toluene.

Herbs

Because of their healing qualities, herbs are useful additions to many natural body care products. They can help increase circulation, reduce inflammation, heal the skin, fight infection, relax the body, and calm the mind. Many herbs have nutrients or antioxidant properties. You can use them by themselves in a bath, face steam, or scrub. You can also make herbs into a tea first and use this as a simple compress by dipping a washcloth into the hot tea, wringing it out, and applying it to the skin. Herbs can be added directly to the bath water in a muslin bag or even an old sock. They make a beautiful addition to natural products such as bath salts, shower scrubs, bath bombs, and body bars.

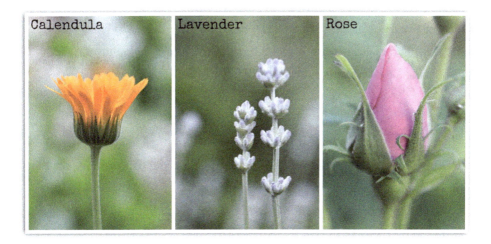

In general, it is better to use dried herbs in any body care product that you are not going to use right away. Fresh herbs are more likely to mold or grow bacteria. Buying dried herbs in a more whole form will keep them fresher for a longer period of time. They often have more visual appeal as well. If necessary, you can powder your herb before making your recipe.

One herb can fall into many categories of herbal actions. There are several categories of actions that are particularly useful for the skin including anti-inflammatories, antimicrobials, astringents, emollients, hemostats, rubefacients, and vulneraries.

Anti-inflammatory herbs

Anti-inflammatory herbs reduce inflammation because they contain various constituents, including salicylates, flavones and precursors to steroids. They are helpful for stings, sprains, contusions, bruises, burns, sore muscles and achy joints. Anti-inflammatory herbs include arnica, aspen, boswellia, chamomile, ginger, licorice, poplar, St. John's wort, turmeric, willow and yucca.

Antimicrobial herbs

Antimicrobial herbs help the body destroy or resist pathogenic microorganisms. They are valuable for infections or the prevention of infection when the skin has been compromised. These herbs include clove, echinacea, garlic, ginger, goldenseal, myrrh, oregano, Oregon grape, sage, thyme, usnea, wormwood and yarrow.

Astringents

Astringent herbs are useful for pulling boggy or inflamed tissues back together. They usually contain tannins, which combine with proteins on the skin to help to tone, tighten, and protect the skin. Astringent herbs tighten pores, helping to reduce potential blemishes and protect the skin from water loss. These herbs include agrimony, bayberry, blackberry, cinnamon, geranium, meadowsweet, oak, plantain, raspberry, rose, rosemary, sage, self-heal, uva ursi, witch hazel and yarrow.

Emollients

Emollient herbs are softening and moistening to the skin. They contain high levels of mucilage making them soothing to dry skin conditions, such as eczema, cracks, and itchy skin. They provide a protective layer for sensitive or mature skin. Aloe vera, chickweed, comfrey, fenugreek, marshmallow, plantain, slippery elm, and violet are emollient, as are fixed oils and butters.

Hemostats

Hemostats help shorten the duration of bleeding by promoting blood clotting or astringing the area. They are useful for wounds and cuts that are bleeding freely. Some hemostats are used internally for the same purposes. They include bayberry, bistort, cayenne, cinnamon, comfrey, geranium, oak, plantain, self-heal, shepherd's purse, turmeric, uva ursi, witch hazel and yarrow.

Rubefacients

Rubefacients cause an increase of circulation to an area by causing capillary dilation. They can be helpful for pain, inflammation, sore joints, achy muscles and tissue repair. Rubefacient herbs include cayenne, cloves, garlic, ginger, horseradish, mustard, nettles, poplar, rosemary, and wintergreen.

Vulneraries

Vulnerary herbs promote skin healing and are useful for wounds, scrapes, scars, skin ulcers, sores and cuts. Vulnerary Herbs include aloe vera, calendula, chickweed, cleavers, comfrey, fenugreek, and plantain.

Here is a list of some of my favorite herbs for the skin. Although most of these herbs can also be used internally, for the purposes of this book, unless otherwise noted, the uses for each herb are for external application. Aloe vera, another favorite herb for the skin, is covered in its own recipe for aloe vera gel.

Aloe (*Aloe barbadensis miller* or *Aloe vera*) Aloe is a wonderfully healing herb for the skin. Its long history of use goes back at least to 4,000 BC when the ancient Egyptians called it the "plant of immortality." It is rich in constituents that are

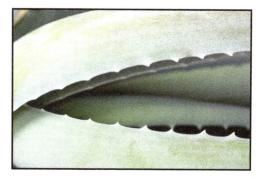

healing for the skin. These include salicylic acid, which is anti-inflammatory and antibacterial, and vitamins A, C and E, which are antioxidants. Aloe also contains glycoproteins, which reduce inflammation, and polysaccharides, which aid skin growth and repair, as well as stimulating immune function.

One of the most useful herbs for the skin, aloe is soothing, cooling and moisturizing. Aloe is useful for dry skin and dandruff. Aloe vera gel or juice stimulates skin growth and repair, making it useful for cuts, burns, wounds, abrasions, skin irritations, scars, stretch marks, and aging skin. It is useful for skin conditions including acne, psoriasis, rashes, sunburn, and herpes.

Aloe is used in products such as lotions, creams, makeup, toothpaste, makeup removers, face toners and shaving creams. An inch of peeled and frozen aloe can be used as a cooling and healing suppository for hemorrhoids. The whole leaves can also be frozen for later use in your recipes.

Calendula (*Calendula officinalis*) Calendula is such a gentle, useful plant, and very easy to grow! It is one of the best herbs for the skin due to its

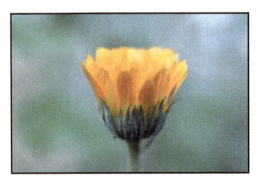

soothing and healing properties. Calendula is antibacterial and antifungal, making it useful for topical infections. It makes an excellent herbal oil, salve, wash, and sitz bath to help heal skin irritations and injuries such as wounds, scratches, bug bites, skin ulcers, rashes, hemorrhoids, diaper rash, and stretch marks. As a vulnerary, it encourages tissue restoration and reduces scarring. This helpful herb can be taken internally or used externally to encourage sweating and is especially useful for eliminating wastes through the skin.

Chamomile (*Matricaria recutita*) Chamomile has been used as a

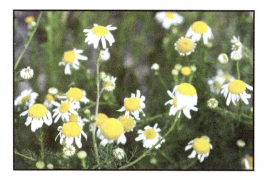

medicinal plant for thousands of years, dating back to the ancient Egyptians, Greeks, and Romans. Chamomile is anti-inflammatory and relaxing. It is helpful for muscle spasms. It makes a good rinse to brighten blond hair. It will help calm frayed nerves and encourage a restful sleep. It is one of my favorite bath herbs for children and babies. This beneficial herb can help to settle the stomach and makes a nice after meal tea.

Comfrey (*Symphytum* spp.) Comfrey is very high in mucilage. Mucilage

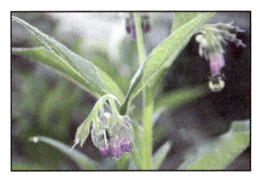

is emollient, making comfrey a wonderfully soothing, moistening, and lubricating plant. As a gargle or mouthwash it will relieve throat infections, hoarseness, or bleeding gums. As a hemostat, comfrey helps stop bleeding. Use a comfrey poultice for sprains and to help repair cartilage, tendon, or ligament damage. Allantoin, a constituent found mainly in comfrey root, is an excellent cell proliferant. It aids healing and new cell growth in wounds, bruises, sores, cuts, burns, skin ulcers, eczema, psoriasis, and varicose veins. Comfrey encourages proper healing to reduce scar tissue. Use it as a poultice or sitz bath to heal perennial tears or hemorrhoids. Comfrey can be used in the bath to soften the skin and makes an excellent herbal oil or healing salve. Be careful when using comfrey with deep wounds as it can encourage tissue growth over the top of the wound before it is properly healed, leading to abscesses. Do not use comfrey internally or on broken skin as the root, and to a lesser degree the leaf, contains pyrrolizidine alkaloids, which may damage the liver with excessive use.

Ginger (*Zingiber officinale*) Ginger is stimulating to the circulatory

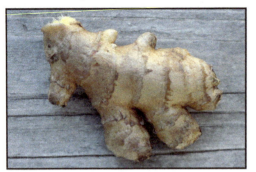

system and encourages sweating. Ginger can be especially helpful for cold and flu-like symptoms. It is a valuable anti-inflammatory, helpful for headaches and painful menstruation. Internally, it aids in digestion and will help to relieve stomach upset, diarrhea, and nausea caused by motion sickness, pregnancy, and the flu. It makes a spicy, warming tea.

Kelp (*Laminaria* spp.)
A highly nutritious sea vegetable, kelp is high in potassium, sodium, calcium, magnesium, zinc, copper, chloride, sulfur, phosphorous, vanadium, cobalt, manganese, selenium, bromine, iodine, arsenic, iron, and fluorine. Its high agar and carrageenan content make it soothing to the skin. It is helpful for muscle and joint pain, and soothing to skin irritations such as eczema and sunburn.

Lavender (*Lavandula* spp.) Lavender is calming for both the skin and

the nerves. It is helpful for burns, sore muscles, tension, headache and bug bites. I like to add this relaxing herb to teas and baths for its soothing effect. It is helpful for easing symptoms of sunburn and itchy, irritated skin. It can be used topically with rashes, eczema, and chickenpox. A bath of the flowers is helpful to ensure a restful night's sleep for both children and adults.

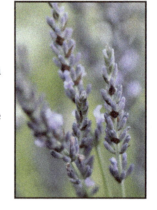

Lemon Balm (*Melissa officinalis*) Lemon balm is uplifting and soothing 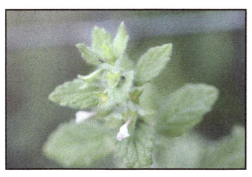 at the same time. Used both internally and externally, it has mild antiviral properties. It is useful for encouraging good cheer, reducing anxiety and perking up a dour demeanor. Lemon balm makes a delightful, nutritive tea that is helpful to calm tension and stress, and encourage a restful sleep.

Mustard (*Brassica* spp.) This pungent little seed is a powerhouse packed with both volatile and fixed oils. Mustard seed is an old remedy for rheumatism, chest congestion, and colds. A mustard pack or a mustard bath helps break up congestion, and encourages sweating by promoting blood flow to the surface of the body. When feeling unwell, you can 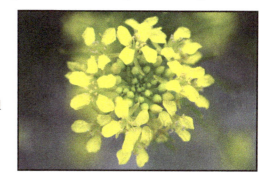 add 1/3 cup powdered mustard seed to a bath. It is useful for fevers, colds, and influenza. As a rubefacient, it will cause mild irritation to the skin, stimulating circulation to that area to relieve muscular and skeletal pain.

Plantain (*Plantago* spp.) A common garden herb, plantain is cooling and 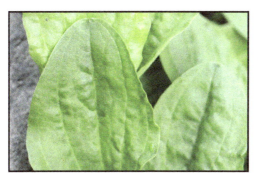 soothing to burns, rashes, sunburn, hives, eczema, psoriasis and chicken pox. It can be used as a tea in a healing bath, poultice or compress applied directly to the skin. High in mucilage, plantain makes a useful, vulnerary compress, oil or salve, helping to heal wounds. It will help draw out a splinter or bee stinger. It is useful for bug bites and nettle stings. Just chew a fresh leaf (dry will work in a pinch) and apply directly to the area. As a hemostat, it will stop bleeding. As an astringent, it is useful for pulling boggy, inflamed tissues back together, allowing for quicker healing.

Rose (*Rosa* spp.) Rose is rejuvenating and slightly astringent to the skin. Touted to help lift the spirits and heal heartache, rose has a loving aroma that is excellent for stress and anxiety. It is anti-inflammatory, antioxidant and antibacterial, making it a healing remedy for the skin wounds, inflammations, infections and injuries. Known as an 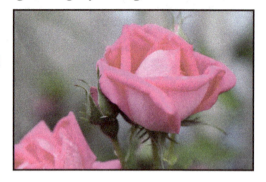 aphrodisiac, rose makes an inviting bath for two. Rose makes a soothing and slightly astringent eye wash. Simply add 30 drops of rose tincture to a 1/2 cup saline solution (1/2 cup warm water and 1/8 teaspoon whole salt—not table salt) and rinse both eyes twice a day. Make this rinse fresh each time you use it.

Rosemary (*Rosmarinus officinalis*) Rosemary is refreshing and 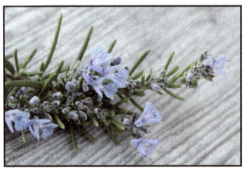 invigorating. It stimulates the mind, encouraging improved memory and concentration. Rosemary makes a wonderful and exhilarating bath, especially stimulating in the morning. It is valuable to ease muscle spasm and head and joint pain. Rosemary encourages circulation. It is said to stimulate hair growth. The tea can be used as a final hair rinse in the shower. Rosemary is antioxidant, helping to eliminate free radicals in the body. Its antimicrobial and antioxidant properties make the extract useful in stabilizing body care products.

Sage (*Salvia officinalis*) Native to the Mediterranean, sage has a long history of use. When taken internally, it aids digestion, and is a traditional cooking herb for meat, stuffing, soup, cheese and sauces. Sage is astringent, making it helpful for reducing swellings and inflammation, including sprains and sore muscles. It is antiseptic and has antimicrobial properties that help fight infection. It is an excellent gargle for sore throat and mouth irritations and infections. Sage is also known for its ability to reduce excessive sweating and makes a useful addition to deodorants for the underarms and feet.

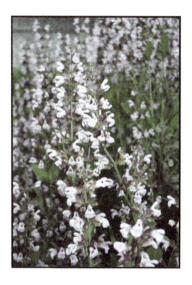

Self-Heal (*Prunella vulgaris*) A common herb, both in the garden and in

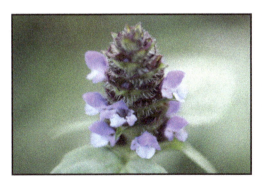

waste areas, self-heal will also grow easily in a lawn. Often the sign of a well-loved herb, it is known by many common names including heart of the earth, heal-all, all-heal, carpenter's herb and hook-heal. It is excellent for the skin. It is astringent, hemostatic, vulnerary, and has mild antiseptic properties. As a hemostat, it will stop bleeding. Self-heal is specific for the mouth and as a mouthwash or gargle it will help to heal inflamed, bleeding gums and skin or mouth ulcers. As an anti-inflammatory, it is useful for insect bites, varicose veins and hemorrhoids. As an antipyretic it may help to reduce a fever. It makes an excellent wash for the eyes. To do this, add 30 drops of self-heal tincture to a

1/2 cup saline solution (1/2 cup warm water and 1/8 teaspoon whole salt – not table salt) and rinse both eyes twice a day. Make this rinse fresh each time you use it.

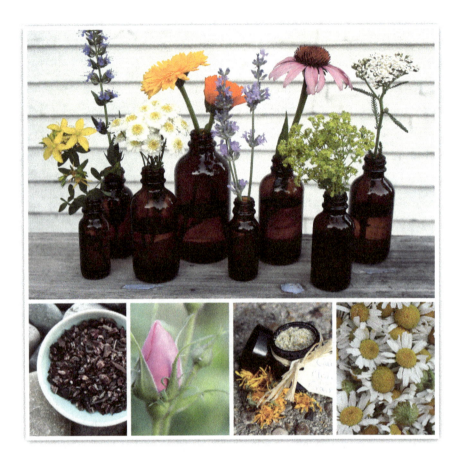

Clays

Clays are naturally occurring, mineral-rich sediments that form a fine powder. They hold water well and pull impurities from the skin as they dry. Clays can be used for the hair, on the skin and as a dry shampoo. Dry shampoos are useful for cleaning the hair without washing away the scalp's natural oils. Clays are also used in various natural body care products including cosmetics, soaps, body powders, creams and lotions. Mixed with water or other liquids, clays can be used as a paste, or mask, over the face, body or a specific organ. The thicker you apply the paste, the longer it takes to dry and the deeper it pulls impurities from the body. Most clays have an indefinite shelf life. Be sure to avoid inhaling clays when working with them as they can irritate the respiratory system.

Dry Clay Shampoo

1) Sprinkle clay in the hair to remove excess oils and impurities.
2) Brush the clay through the hair and allow to sit 5-10 minutes.
3) Turn the head upside down over a sink, bathtub or trashcan and brush out the residual clay.

Bentonite clay

Also called montmorillonite, bentonite clay can be used both externally and internally in small amounts to remove waste products, toxins and skin impurities. I use it for more medicinal purposes on the skin, for spider bites, abcesses and bee stings. It is commonly used in facial masks, body powders, lotions, creams and cosmetics. The largest bentonite deposits come from the United States, specifically Wyoming and Montana. Bentonite is a unique clay in that it is a naturally occurring byproduct of volcanic ash exposed to windy and wet weather conditions. High in silicon dioxide, calcium oxide and aluminum oxide, bentonite should be a grayish cream color, not bright white.

Fuller's earth

Fuller's earth has many names, most of which are quite descriptive of how it is best used, including bleaching or whitening clay, oil absorption clay and earth clay. With a long history of use, the name Fuller comes from the term for workers who once used the clay to absorb excess lanolin from sheep's wool. Off white in appearance, Fuller's earth is highly absorbent. Found throughout the world, it excels in soaking up oils and other materials and is used both in the automotive industry and as a kitty litter ingredient. It is the best clay for oily skin and is useful for acne and skin blemishes. Fuller's earth is used as a body powder, dry shampoo, facial mask and herbal body pack. Chemically referred to as magnesium aluminum silicate, it is composed mainly of alumina, silica, iron oxides, lime, and magnesium, in variable proportions. Make sure to avoid industrial Fuller's earth from an auto supply stores. Go for the good stuff by purchasing from reputable herb and body care suppliers!

Green clay

Green clay, also called sea clay, is more nourishing to the skin than other clays as it contains plant material. It also contains montmorillonite, mineral oxides, magnesium, calcium, potassium, dolomite, silica, manganese, phosphorous, silicon, copper, and selenium. Green clay is used to lighten skin and to absorb excess oil. This clay was originally mined in France, but is also found in Europe and the northwestern U.S. It is commonly used as a facemask for dry or sensitive skin and works well applied to insect bites and rashes. The clay should be green to light green in color.

Kaolin

Kaolin, also called white cosmetic clay, is good for all skin types. It is useful as a general, all-purpose clay for cosmetics, powders, body and facemasks, skin care products, and deodorants. Kaolin is the most commonly used clay in cosmetics because of its light, fine texture. It consists of iron, magnesium, calcium, sodium, zinc, and kaolinite, a silicate mineral found in abundance in the Earth's crust all over the globe.

Red clay

Red clay, also called Moroccan, ghassoul, oxide or rhassoul clay, is drying and absorbent. It is especially good for oily or problem skin and can help tighten pores. Historically used for body wraps in Turkish baths, it contains dolomite, silica, ferric oxide (a type of iron, which gives it its red hue), calcium, magnesium, potassium, sodium and mineral oxides.

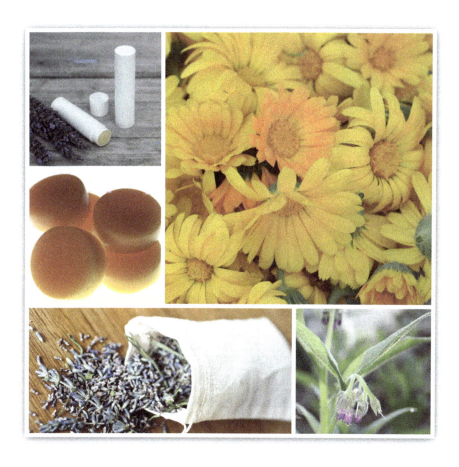

Natural Colorants

Natural colorants can add pigment and visual appeal to body care products and bath salts. Many of the natural ingredients listed below have their own healing properties. I recommend staying away from artificial food coloring and other synthetic colorants as they can irritate the skin and nervous system.

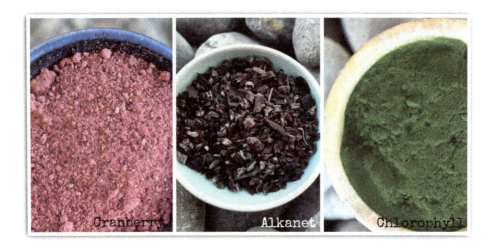

Alkanet (*Alkanna tinctoria*)
Alkanet root is primarily used as a dying and coloring agent, especially for fabrics, soap, lip balm, lipstick and wood. It imparts a red to pinkish color. Alkanet is insoluble in water but can be easily extracted into alcohol or oil. It is soothing and astringent to irritated skin. Because it contains pyrrolizidine alkaloids, which can be harmful to the liver, do not apply alkanet to broken or abraded skin.

Annatto (*Bixa orellana*)
Annatto seeds provide a beautiful red hue. Popular over the centuries as a body paint in South America, now annatto is commonly used to color margarine and cheese. It is antibacterial and slightly astringent to the skin. Annatto is good for blisters and mouth sores. It contains powerful

carotenoids, which act as potent antioxidants to protect the skin from free radical damage.

Beet (*Beta vulgaris*)

Beet powder not only adds a lovely pink tone to a body care or bath product, it is also highly nutritious. Beets are high in vitamin C, iron, magnesium, folate, manganese, potassium, copper and fiber. Some of the phytonutrients in beets, called betalains, have excellent antioxidant, anti-inflammatory and antifungal properties. Many years ago, women would rub their cheeks with fresh beets, improving their complexion and adding a pink hue to the skin as a natural blush. Beets can also be used as an ingredient in face toners, masks, and as a natural dye mixed with henna to provide auburn highlights.

Cacao (*Theobroma cacao*)

Cacao is the main ingredient in chocolate. Its Latin name means "food of the gods." Constituents of cacao, including phenethylamine, encourage feelings of pleasure and wellbeing. No wonder so many people like chocolate! It has antioxidant properties, in particular flavanols, which reduce free radical damage and protect from UV light. Cacao encourages skin suppleness and hydration. Cacao powder and cocoa butter are both from *Theobroma cacao* and make a nice combination used together. Using the pure, powdered cacao bean is best and will impart a rich brown color to salts, scrubs and facemasks.

Chlorophyll

Chlorophyll is the primary light-absorbing pigment, deep green in color, which initiates photosynthesis in green plants. Interestingly, the chlorophyll molecule is chemically similar to human blood except that its central atom is magnesium, whereas human blood's is iron. I feel this makes chlorophyll uniquely beneficial to the human body. It is extremely nutritive, being high in minerals, most notably magnesium, and vitamins. It is antioxidant, anti-inflammatory and anti-microbial. Functioning as a skin protectant against oxidative damage, chlorophyll is often found in creams, lotions and serums that are meant to prevent wrinkles and fine lines. It is also used in soaps, body sprays, deodorants, mouthwashes, toothpastes, and breath fresheners. Chlorophyll is useful for acne, blemishes and breakouts. In its pure form it is only soluble in oil. Be warned that a little chlorophyll goes a long way.

Cranberry (*Vaccinium* spp.)

Cranberry adds a beautiful pink color to natural body care products and bath salts. It is healing to the skin, antioxidant, and astringent making it useful as a toner for oily skin. Proanthocyanidin, a plant constituent found in cranberries, inhibits the growth of bacteria, making it useful to prevent plaque buildup in the mouth as well as aiding acne, boils, pimples, problem skin and urinary tract infections. It is high in vitamins C, B3, and B5 and will help to firm the skin and reduce the appearance of wrinkles, redness, skin pigmentation and fine lines. Enzymes present in this fruit are useful for exfoliating dead skin cells. Cranberry is good for the scalp and hair and will aid in the treatment of dandruff and psoriasis. Cranberry contains salicylic acid, also found in aspirin, making it useful to alleviate inflammation, aches, and pains.

Mineral Oxides

Mineral Oxides are natural mineral pigments from the earth. They come in many different colors and you can blend them together to create your own shades. They are used for making mineral make up, soaps and other natural body care products. Start with small amounts and increase as needed. Warning: it can impart a color to your bathtub, bowls, kitchen utensils, etc. making additional cleaning necessary. Make sure any mineral oxide that you buy is safe for your intended application such as the eyes or lips. The intended applications should be listed with the product. A caution: a little mineral oxide goes a long way in coloring a product.

Turmeric (*Curcuma longa*)

A common cooking spice, turmeric has been used as a natural body care agent in India for centuries. It is traditionally used for acne, dark spots on the skin, exfoliation, stretch marks and burns. It has anti-inflammatory, antibacterial and anti-aging properties. Turmeric is very yellow, which can add vibrant color to any body care product. Be cautious where you put it, however, as it can temporarily stain the skin and various kitchen or bath surfaces. Kasturi turmeric (*Curcuma aromatica*) is nonstaining and inedible, but more difficult to find outside India.

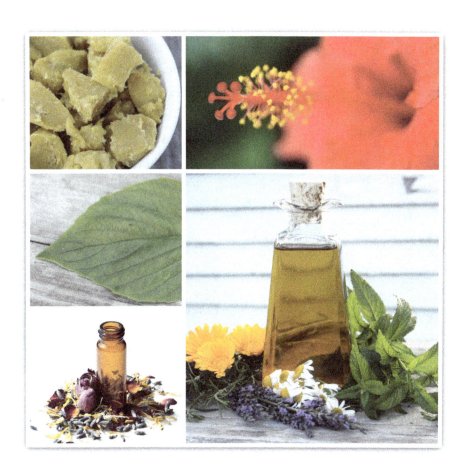

Essential Oils

Essential oils add aroma and other healing properties to body care products. Many essential oils are also antimicrobial and act as mild preservatives. Some of my favorite oils for the skin and body are listed below, and there are many more to choose from. While true essential oils are therapeutic and healing to the body and mind, synthetic fragrances are not effective in the same way. Synthetic fragrances can sometimes irritate skin and mucus membranes, and some are even neurotoxins. These chemicals actually function as a form of air pollution and can be counterproductive when added to natural products. Stick with the good stuff!

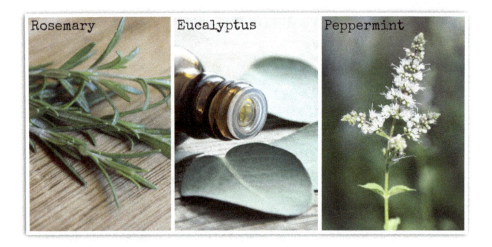

Essential oils are extremely potent and should almost always be diluted before using them on the body. To do this, you can add them to salt, herbs, butters, fixed oils, vinegar, honey, yogurt or milk. To get the greatest healing benefit in a bath, I recommend getting into the bath first and then adding your bath blend. Please remember that essential oils are recommended for external use only; they are generally too strong to be ingested. If you are pregnant, nursing, have health concerns or are using essential oils with babies or children, please research your oils before using them.

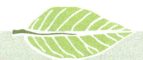

Common recommendations for diluting essential oils

- 1 milliliter (mL) of essential oil is equal to 30-40 drops, depending on the viscosity. The thicker the oil, the larger each drop will be. Larger drops will cause fewer drops to be in a milliliter.

- 1%: 5-6 drops per ounce of carrier oil or body care product. Children, pregnant women, the elderly, those who are very sick and sensitive people should use this dilution. It is also a good dilution for face care products.

- 2%: 10-12 drops per ounce of carrier oil or body care product is the most common dilution. It is used for most natural skin care recipes.

- 7-10 %: 35-60 drops per ounce of carrier oil or body care product. This dilution is used for areas of specific application, such as an infection on the skin.

Birch (*Betula* spp.)

Birch is excellent for body aches and pains such as sore muscles, tendons, and joints. It is pain relieving, anti-inflammatory and imparts a warming sensation. Use birch for sprains, arthritis, tired or sore muscles, and before or after working out. It is also helpful for dandruff and psoriasis. Caution: if you are taking blood thinners or have trouble with blood clotting, avoid birch as it contains methyl salicylate, which thins the blood.

Cedar (*Cedrus* spp.)
Atlas cedar relieves congestion, coughs and sore muscles. Cedar will help reduce oily skin, acne and dandruff. It is said to be one of the best oils for cellulite. Cedar has a calming, relaxing and grounding affect.

Cinnamon (*Cinnamomum* spp.)
Cinnamon is a potent antioxidant, helping to preserve natural products and destroy free radicals that can prematurely age the skin. It is excellent for relieving pain and is warming upon application. It is one of the best antimicrobial oils and is a potent antibacterial, antiviral and antifungal. Cinnamon is a delicious and effective ingredient in toothpastes or powders.

Eucalyptus (*Eucalyptus radiata*)
Eucalyptus can be especially beneficial when fighting colds, flu and coughs. It helps to clear congestion and can relieve muscle and joint pain. Eucalyptus is cooling and anti-inflammatory. It is helpful for acne and problem skin. There are many other species of eucalyptus essential oils so make sure you research each one for its unique healing properties before use.

Geranium (*Pelargonium gravolens*)
Geranium is also known as rose geranium. It is a wonderful balancer for the hormones, and the body in general. Geranium has both antifungal and antibacterial properties. It is useful for eczema, cellulite, acne, burns, stretch marks and overall tissue repair. It can be used on all skin types.

Lavender (*Lavandula* spp.)
Lavender essential oil is my number-one first aid remedy. It can be used full strength on most people's skin for burns, infections, bug bites and stings, and skin inflammation and irritation. It is helpful for pain and headaches as well as being soothing for emotional upset or insomnia. Keep a spray bottle filled with lavender in your medicine cabinet, purse or first aid kit. Since my children were babies, I have sprayed it on their scrapes and injuries. I often spray it on a bandage before applying it to a scraped knee or elbow. It has an amphoteric action, meaning it can be relaxing or stimulating based on

dilution. In small amounts lavender is quite relaxing, and in large amounts it is stimulating. Lavender can also help to boost the body's natural immune response. Before using it full strength, do a patch test first by applying a small amount to the skin and watching for redness or irritation. Some people find that too much lavender will bring on a headache.

Marjoram (*Origanum majorana*)

Marjoram is relaxing and calming. It is excellent oil for sore muscles and will ease muscle spasms, menstrual cramps, headaches and stiff or sore joints. Marjoram will help to heal the skin and is useful for bug bites, bruises, burns and both fungal and bacterial infections.

Orange (*Citrus sinensis*)

Orange is antiseptic, calming, refreshing and uplifting. It is good for nervousness, stress and tension. Orange is also useful to alleviate water retention, move the lymph and to soothe cold and flu symptoms. It is helpful for overall detoxification, increasing circulation and is useful to reduce cellulite. Orange is good for acne and oily hair and skin. Caution: citrus oils can be photosensitizing and should not be used on the skin when in the sun.

Peppermint (*Mentha piperita*)

Peppermint is helpful for digestion, nausea and motion sickness. Highly antimicrobial, it is useful for fighting bacterial, viral and parasitic infections. Peppermint helps to reduce pain, sore joints and stiff muscles. It is uplifting, stimulating and encourages focus. Peppermint is cooling, making a refreshing addition to toothpaste or a footbath. It is an excellent remedy for headaches and combines well with lavender or eucalyptus for this purpose.

Rose (*Rosa centifolia, R. damascena*)

Rose is considered a precious essential oil, meaning it is expensive and labor intensive to manufacture. A rose blossom contains only around 0.02% essential oil, so it takes an average of 60,000 roses to produce just 1 ounce of oil. Rose is one of the finest essential oils for the skin. Appropriate for all skin types, it is antioxidant, anti-inflammatory, emollient, and healing to the skin.

It is excellent for mature skin, fine lines and wrinkles. Rose is balancing, astringent, and antiseptic. It has mild anti-viral and bactericidal properties.

Rosemary (*Rosmarinus officinalis*)

Rosemary is particularly valuable for alleviating symptoms of respiratory infections, colds, flu and bronchitis. It is antiseptic and antioxidant. Rosmarinic acid, which is derived from rosemary, is often used to preserve body care products. A stimulating aroma, it offers a refreshing boost to ward off physical and mental fatigue. It is valuable for sore muscles and joints, varicose veins, and hair loss prevention.

Tea Tree (*Melaleuca alternifolia*)

Tea tree is antifungal, antibacterial, and antiviral and works to stimulate the body's natural immune defenses during a cold or flu. It can help to combat both yeast and bacterial infections, and is a healing oil for vaginal infections. It makes a lovely footbath or toothpaste ingredient. Tea tree is helpful for oily skin, acne, skin blemishes, sunburn, insect bites and dandruff. It is one of the only essential oils that can be used undiluted on the skin for most people. Tea tree could find a home in most people's medicine cabinets or first aid kits.

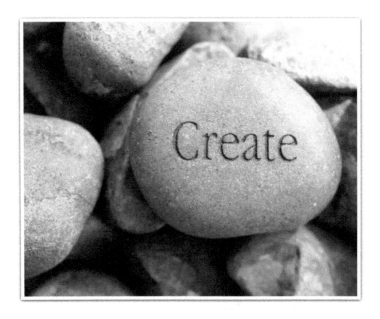

Natural Salts

The foundation of any bath salt is, of course, salt. For a truly healing bath experience, I prefer to stay away from table salt, which has been processed to remove trace elements and contains anti-caking agents and other undesirable additives. Instead, try some of the salts recommended below. Salts can usually be found in different grinds, from fine to corase, or larger. I prefer a fine grind if you will be rubbing it on the skin, such as a body scrub. A coarse grind can make an attractive bath salt. Deposits of salt can also include pollutants from the air, chemicals from rain that fell on the deposits, and elements from soil surrounding the water or deposits. According to the National Center for Ecological Analysis and Synthesis, some of the cleanest ocean water, and therefore the purest sea salt, is found in the following areas: Australia, Belize, Grenada, Tonga, Samoa, Qatar, British Pacific Territories and Russia.

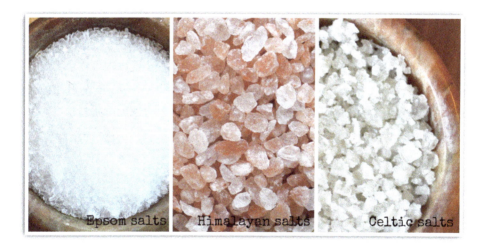

Celtic sea salts
Celtic salts have a natural balance of minerals and trace elements from the ocean. These salts are traditionally hand-harvested in Guérande, France, in the Brittany region. Their gray color results from the salt's natural trace minerals absorbed from the sea. Unwashed, unrefined, and additive-free, this

salt contains many minerals vital to the human body such as calcium, potassium, copper, zinc and iron. This salt is lower in sodium than table salt.

Dead Sea salts

Differing greatly from other sea salts in mineral content, Dead Sea salts made up of only 12–18% sodium chloride with a high percentage of chloride, bromide, magnesium, calcium and potassium. They are valued for their healing properties for arthritis, skin conditions and allergies.

Epsom salt

Epsom salt gets its name from the town of Epsom in England where it was originally discovered. It is a pure mineral compound of magnesium sulfate in crystal form. Epsom salt is healing to sprains and bruises, relaxes sore muscles, draws impurities out of the skin, and is mildly astringent. Magnesium sulfate is absorbed through the skin, and taking an Epsom salt bath is a safe and easy way to increase sulfate and magnesium levels in the body.

Hawaiian red salt

Hawaiian Red salt is a natural, unprocessed salt. It gets its distinctive color from purified red Hawaiian clay. Volcanic red clay is high in iron oxide, and can be useful in healing wounds, body aches, and muscle sprains. It is believed to draw toxins from overworked muscles.

Himalayan salt

Himalayan salt contains many valuable trace elements. These salts have a beautiful, natural pink coloring that makes them a perfect option for attractive, colorful bath salts. Himalayan salt can be purchased in large chunks called "rocks." Larger rocks can be used in the bath several times before they dissolve completely.

Sea salt

Astringent and antiseptic, a finely ground sea salt makes an effective and inexpensive body scrub. Sea salt is often evaporated from the ocean instead of excavated in salt mines. Every ocean source has different trace mineral composition and a unique flavor profile. Trace minerals in sea salt include sulfate, magnesium, calcium, potassium, bicarbonate, bromide, borate, strontium, and fluoride.

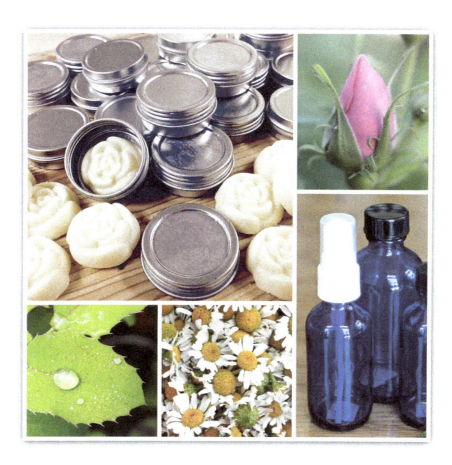

Fixed Oils

Fixed oils are natural, non-volatile oils derived from fruits, vegetables, nuts and seeds. Often called carrier oils, they do not evaporate like essential oils. Fixed oils are a main ingredient in many natural body care recipes. They help moisturize, lubricate and protect the skin. Whenever possible, use cold pressed, unrefined oils as they are more nourishing to the skin.

Rancid oils should be avoided as they contain free radicals, which might increase the risk of developing diseases such as cancer or heart disease. Rancid oils can also cause inflammation. There are several ways to tell if an oil is rancid. Firstly, the smell is "off." Some people describe them as having the smell of crayons or rancid nuts. The texture feels greasy or even tacky. Lastly, I have noticed that the colors of some rancid oils such as olive oil turn lighter. This is even true for products that turn rancid such as salves.

There are a few best practices for handling fixed oils and maximizing their shelf life. It is generally best to store fixed oils in airtight containers in the refrigerator, or in a dark, cool cabinet. On the label of each oil, write the date purchased and the expected shelf life. Keep lids on tightly, and don't have extra room in oil bottles as air causes oils to oxidize. Following are a few of my favorite fixed oils. There are many more to choose from.

Almond oil (*Prunus dulcis*)
A medium-consistency oil useful by itself for massage, almond oil is a nice base for other oils. It is good for most skin types and makes an excellent makeup remover. It is rich in vitamin E and oleic and linoleic acids. Useful for psoriasis and eczema, almond oil is also good for hair and scalp health. It has a shelf life of about 1 year.

Avocado oil (*Persea americana*)
Avocado oil is a thick, rich oil. It can be diluted with other carrier oils to thin the consistency. Avocado oil is high in vitamins A, B1, B2, D, and E as well as

amino acids, sterols, pantothenic acid, lecithin, and other essential fatty acids. It is excellent for mature skin, psoriasis, eczema and sensitive or problem skin. Store this oil in the refrigerator. Avocado's shelf life is about 1 year.

Grape seed oil (*Vitis vinifera*)
Grape seed oil is odorless, light in texture, and is easily absorbed by the skin. It is softening and soothing, making it an ideal skincare and cosmetic ingredient. It is good for oily skin as it is a thinner oil with mildly astringent properties. Grape seed oil contains proanthocyanidins, which are considered to be very potent antioxidants, making it helpful for reducing the sun's damaging effects and decreasing free-radical damage to the skin. It has a shelf life of about 6 months to 1 year.

Hazelnut oil (*Corylus avellana*)
Hazelnut oil is light and astringent, making it truly excellent for oily and acne prone skin. It absorbs quickly and encourages skin elasticity and cell regeneration. This oil is often used as a base oil for essential oils. It has a shelf life of about 1 year.

Jojoba (*Simmondsia chinensis*)
Technically not an oil, jojoba is a wax that is liquid at room temperature. Because of its extremely long shelf life, it is my top choice for mixing with precious essential oils. One of my favorite oils for the skin, jojoba is chemically very similar to sebum, the oil our skin produces. It is good for dry skin and dandruff. It is extremely stable and can last many years without going rancid.

Neem oil (*Azadirachta indica*)
Neem is antibacterial, antifungal, and antimicrobial. It is wonderful for skin infections, acne and eczema. Diluted, it makes an effective insect repellant, and can be sprayed on plants as a natural pesticide. Neem has a strong odor and is very dark in color. It has a shelf life of about 2 years.

Olive oil (*Olea europaea*)

Olive oil has a long history of use for the skin. It has been used for massage, and as a skin cleanser and moisturizer. It is antioxidant and contains linoleic acid, an essential fatty acid that is moisturizing to the skin. I like to use it in lotions and salves. I recommend using extra virgin olive oil as it has more nutrients for the skin and is more stable. It has a shelf life of 2–3 years.

Rosehip seed oil (*Rosa* spp.)

Rosehip seed oil is full of vitamins, antioxidants and Omega-3 and 6 fatty acids. A very light, non-greasy oil, it is helpful in reducing dark spots and hydrating dry, itchy skin. Rosehip seed oil is good for dermatitis, acne and eczema. It supports mature skin and is great for wrinkles, scars and fine lines. Rosehip seed oil is fragile and has a shelf life of approximately 6 months. Be sure to store it in the refrigerator.

Sea Buckthorn oil (*Hippophae rhamnoides*)

Sea Buckthorn oil is high in antioxidants, vitamins C, A, and E, beta-carotene, minerals, amino acids, and essential fatty acids. It is used medicinally both internally and topically. High in Omega-3 oils, it is helpful for mature skin, sunburn, eczema, and healing wounds. Use it for acne, dermatitis, skin inflammation, dry skin, and skin ulcers. It is very orange in color and can stain clothing. It is generally used as a small part of a recipe. It has a shelf life of 1 year.

Sesame oil (*Sesamum indicum*)

Sesame oil is high in Vitamin E and antioxidants. It offers mild, natural sun protection. Sesame oil is used in Ayurvedic medicine to reduce stress-related symptoms. It is a thicker oil and is helpful for dry skin, eczema, psoriasis, and dandruff. Sesame oil has a shelf life of 2 years and should be stored in the refrigerator.

Walnut oil (*Juglans* spp.)

Rich in Omega-3 essential fatty acid, walnut oil is ideal for body massage and can be used as nutrient-rich addition to any lotion or body oil. It is anti-inflammatory and antioxidant making it valuable for mature, dry or damaged skin. This oil is best stored in the refrigerator. The shelf life is about 1 year.

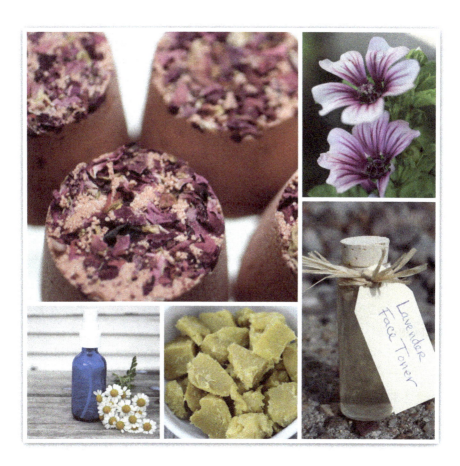

Butters

Butters differ from oils in that they are solid at room temperature. They tend to be highly moisturizing and nourishing to the skin. Butters help thicken a recipe and enhance the natural skin barrier existing between us and our environment.

When using butters in a recipe, small beads or bumps may develop. This is known as crystallization, or graininess. You are more likely to get graininess in your recipes from using unrefined butters than refined or ultra-refined butters. It is also important to note that the more unrefined, also called virgin, a butter is, the more nutrients and healing properties it will contain. I prefer to put up with occasional graininess in a recipe than miss out on the healing properties of an unrefined butter.

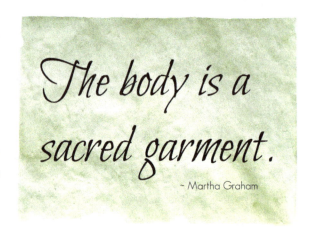

The body is a sacred garment.
~ Martha Graham

Tempering Butters:

There are several ways to reduce graininess when using butters. Sometimes tempering the butter can help. To do this, heat it to 175° F (80° C) in a double boiler. Then cool the butter to about 70° F (21° C). You can also try heating the butter and then cooling it quickly in the refrigerator or freezer. Sometimes heating the butter very slowly over low heat can help. If you do get graininess in a recipe, not to worry; most butters will melt on contact with the skin.

Carnauba wax (*Copernicia cerifera*)

Carnauba wax is a natural vegetable wax exuded by the leaves of a palm tree, which grows in Brazil. It is the hardest natural wax available, so a little goes a long way. It is emollient, moisturizing, and helps to protect the skin. Use it to make creams, salves, ointments, protective creams, balms, pomades, lipsticks, mascaras and lip gloss. It is a good substitute for beeswax and is especially helpful if you are trying to make a vegan salve or lip balm. There is conflicting information about whether using carnauba wax may contribute to the damage of tropical rainforests. Make sure you are getting your wax from an ethically grown and harvested source. It is soluble in alcohol and fixed oils, and is insoluble in water. It has a high melting point (about 176° F or 80° C), so melt the wax well before incorporating it into your formula. Use it as 2–40% of your recipe, depending on the hardness desired.

Cocoa butter (*Theobroma cacao*)

Made from the cacao bean, this butter is hard at room temperature but will melt on contact with the skin. It is a natural antioxidant and moisturizer and is good for treating dry or irritated skin and stretch marks. It is an excellent addition to lotions, creams, salves, lip balm and body butters. Best of all, it smells like chocolate! The melting point for cocoa butter is around 93° F (34° C). It is very stable, with a shelf life of 2–3 years.

Coconut oil (*Cocos nucifera*)

Coconut oil is over 90% saturated fat. It has antimicrobial, antibacterial, and antifungal properties. It makes an amazing hair de-frizzer, body scrubber, and makeup remover. It is useful in recipes such as lip balms, salves, and lotions. It is antioxidant and absorbs quickly into the skin. Virgin coconut oil has the lovely smell of coconuts and is my favorite type for the skin and to use in food. One of the softer butters, coconut oil has a melting point of about 76° F (24° C). It is very stable, with a shelf life 2–4+ years.

Cupuacu butter (*Theobroma grandiflorum*)

Related to the cacao tree, cupuacu butter contains essential fatty acids and phytosterols that make it very moisturizing for the skin and hair. It provides natural protection from UV-A and UV-B rays. It is helpful for skin conditions such as eczema and dermatitis and adds shine and moisture to hair. It is emollient, moisturizing and encourages elasticity and water retention in the skin. It is used in salves, lip balms, creams, foot balms, lotions and hair care products. Cupuacu butter can be used as a non-hydrogenated replacement for stearic acid in a recipe. It is one of the softer butters with a creamy consistency. It has a low melting point of about 86° F (30° C) and can help soften a formula that contains harder butters or waxes. It has a shelf life of about 2 years.

Kokum butter (*Garcinia indica*)

Originating in India, kokum butter is somewhat dry, hard and cracked in appearance. It melts on contact with the skin. Kokum butter is high in fatty acids and antioxidants. Kokum Butter helps regenerate the skin and its emollient properties encourage flexibility and softness. Use it for rough, dry, calloused skin and feet. It is useful for skin inflammation and irritation such as rashes and eczema. It is valuable in salves, lotions, ointments, butters and creams. Use kokum butter in small amounts mixed with fixed oils and softer butters. The melting point for Kokum is approximately 100° F (38° C). To prevent graininess, temper this butter by heating it to 175° F (80° C) in a double boiler. Then cool the butter to about 70° F (21° C). Kokum butter has a shelf life of about 2 years.

Mango butter (*Mangifera indica*)

Mango butter has natural skin-softening properties and is deeply moisturizing. Due to its regenerative properties, it is good for mature skin, wrinkles, fine lines, dry skin and for healing wounds. It is a harder butter and is best added to softer butters or fixed oils. It makes a wonderful addition to salves, lotions, lip balms, and body scrubs. It is helpful to temper the butter by heating it to around 150° F (65° C) before adding it to your recipe. It has a melting point of around 90° F (32° C) and a shelf life is about 1 year.

Shea butter (*Vitellaria paradoxa*, but this tree nut is often referred to by its old name of *Butyrospermum parkii*)

Shea butter is also called karite butter and is made from the nuts of the African karite nut tree. It melts on contact and is readily absorbed into the skin, without leaving a greasy residue. It is nutrient rich, containing vitamins A and E, as well as catechins, plant antioxidants also found in green tea. Shea butter is anti-inflammatory. High in fatty acids, it will soften dry skin and brittle hair. You can make a simple whipped body butter by heating shea butter it until it is soft and mixing it in a mixer for about 5 minutes. Refrigerate it for 15 minutes, and mix it again until it has a light and fluffy consistency. The fresher you are able to get this butter, the better. Shea butter can be particularly grainy. Tempering can help to avoid this; heat the butter to 175° F (80° C) for 20 minutes before using. The shelf life of Shea butter is 1–2 years.

Natural Thickeners

Natural thickeners help to emulsify oil and water-based ingredients together so they form a stable mixture. They are particularly helpful when making lotions, creams, creamy cleansers and serums, which are skin care products that have a high concentration of active ingredients. Natural thickeners help improve the consistency of a recipe and often provide healing properties of their own. Different thickeners are suitable for different applications and mix best with either the oil or water-based ingredients in your recipe.

Acacia gum (*Acacia* spp.)
Also known as gum arabic, acacia is derived from the stems and branches of the Acacia tree in Africa. It contains various polysaccharides such as glucuronic and galacturonic acids that are beneficial to the skin. This powder should be added to water ingredients in a formula and will help to preserve your recipe. It can best be used in creams, lotions, balms, pomades, shampoos, body washes, makeup and gels. Use as 1–10 % of your recipe.

Arrowroot (*Maranta arundinacea*)
Native to the West Indies and Central and South America, arrowroot is a starch derived from the tuber of the plant. It gives a smooth feeling to the skin and is demulcent and emollient. It can be used as a body powder, in a deodorant, or in the bath. It can be added to lotions and creams to help moisturizers absorb and make the lotion less greasy. I like to use it as a replacement in any recipe that calls for cornstarch. Add it to the water-based ingredients in your formula. Use as 2% of a recipe.

Beeswax
A glandular excretion from bees, beeswax is extremely stable and will never go rancid. It is very protective for the skin. Melt it first and mix it with the oil-based ingredients in your recipe. Use it to thicken creams, lotions, pomades, salves, ointments, lip balms, lipsticks, mascara, foundations, eye shadows,

cold creams, lotions and creams. Add beeswax to the oil-based ingredients in your recipe. Use it as 2–40% of your recipe.

Carnauba wax (*Copernicia cerifera*)

Carnauba wax is a natural vegetable wax exuded by the leaves of a palm tree, which grows in Brazil. It is the hardest natural wax available, so a little goes a long way. It is emollient, moisturizing, and helps to protect the skin. Use it to make creams, salves, ointments, protective creams, balms, pomades, lipsticks, mascaras and lip gloss. It is a good substitute for beeswax for those that prefer vegan body care products. It is soluble in alcohol and fixed oils, and is insoluble in water. It has a high melting point (about 176° F or 80° C), so melt the wax well before incorporating it into your formula. Use it as 2–40% of your recipe, depending on the hardness desired.

> *There are days I drop words of comfort on myself like falling leaves and remember that it is enough to be taken care of by myself.* ~ Brian Andreas

Cornstarch (*Zea mays*)

Cornstarch softens and calms itchy skin. It makes a useful body powder ingredient. It can be added to lotions to help moisturizers absorb and make the lotion less greasy. Make sure to purchase non-genetically modified corn products, also called non-GMO (genetically modified organism). Cornstarch should be added to the water part of a recipe. Use as 2% of a formula.

Guar gum (*Cyamopsis tetragonolobus*)

Derived from the seeds of the guar plant, it is conditioning to the skin and hair and can be used in shampoos, conditioners, lotions, creams, body washes and shower gels. Guar gum should be mixed with an acidic water base that has a pH of 7 or more. You can use a pH strip to test this. You can attain this by adding citric acid or lemon juice to your water mixture. Use as .2–2% of a formula.

Lecithin

Lecithin is a mixture of phospholipids and oils. It can be derived from many sources including soybeans, eggs, milk, and many nuts and seeds including sunflower seeds and rapeseed (canola). Most commonly derived from soybeans, it can be made from genetically modified crops. It is available as either a powder or liquid. Lecithin is softening to the skin and can be used to both thicken body care products and help preserve them. If you have a soy allergy, I recommend choosing another thickener or making sure of your source by talking to the manufacturer. Add lecithin to the oil part of your recipe. It can be used at 1–2% dilution.

Stearic acid

Made from a fatty acid naturally occurring in vegetables, stearic acid is helpful for making soaps, creams, lotions, and shaving creams. Although very easy to work with, stearic acid is hydrogenated, making it more refined and less desirable than many other natural body care ingredients listed in this book. It is oil and alcohol-soluble and should be added to the oil part of your mixture. Warm it to incorporate it into your oils. Use it as 2 - 10% of your recipe.

Xanthan gum

Xanthan gum is a natural polysaccharide used in food and cosmetics as a thickener and stabilizer. It is made by a fermentation process with the bacteria *Xanthomonas campestris* with carbohydrates from corn, wheat, dairy or soy. Xanthan gum is hydrating to the skin. Slowly sprinkle it into the water-based ingredients in your recipe and let it incorporate for approximately 15 minutes, whisking vigorously until smooth. Use as .1–1% of a formula.

Other Natural Products for the Skin

Many foods and other natural products can be used on the skin. Most of these ingredients have their own healing properties and many of them are edible. It is helpful to know that an ingredient is safe to put on the skin if it is healthy to ingest. These are a few of my favorite ingredients. You may already have many of these in your kitchen, while some of them are more likely found in an herb or health food store.

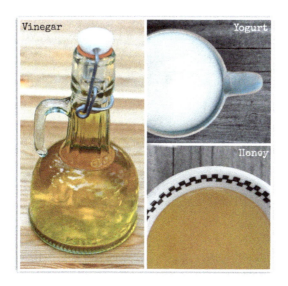

Apple cider vinegar

Apple cider vinegar has a pH of about 4.5 to 5.5, which is very similar to the skin. I recommend purchasing raw, organic, unfiltered apple cider vinegar and always diluting it before applying it to the body. Mix 1 part apple cider vinegar with 2 parts water to make a face toner that will help to restore a more balanced pH and gently exfoliate the skin. It can increase sensitivity to ultraviolet rays so it is best applied at night before bed. It is useful for acne, warts and sunburn. Apple cider vinegar makes a wonderful hair rinse, will help lighten dark spots on skin, and is a good antifungal agent. In the bath, it softens water by making minerals more soluble and can be used to break up essential oil drops and incorporate them into the bath.

Baking soda

Also called sodium bicarbonate, baking soda is both alkalinizing and exfoliating. It is mildly antiseptic and will help prevent infections. Baking soda is valuable as a deodorant, toothpaste, and shampoo. It is useful in a bath to help relieve sunburn and can be helpful when applied to skin funguses. After using baking soda, make sure to rinse it off with water and then do a vinegar rinse of 1 part apple cider vinegar to 2 parts water to restore proper pH balance to the skin and hair.

Borax

Borax is a natural, alkaline mineral that cleans without drying the skin. It can be found in the detergent section of the grocery store (make sure you are getting PURE borax). It has emulsifying properties that improve the consistency of creams and lotions, especially when using beeswax. Borax is highly alkaline and should only be used in small amounts. For making a lotion or cream, add it to the liquid part of your formula. It should be about 1% of the recipe.

Fruits and Vegetables

Vegetables and fruits are often useful for skin care. Many contain antioxidants and enzymes that help to restore the skin. Some that are notable include avocado, blueberries, bananas, papayas, and strawberries. Citrus fruits are also wonderful for the hair and skin, but don't use them when you will be in the sun, as citrus oils can cause an increased risk of sunburn (called photosensitization) and eventual dark spots on the skin.

Honey

Honey is made from bees gathering flower nectar, partially digesting it, and then evaporating it down into the thick and golden concoction that we know as honey. An effective humectant, honey draws water to the skin. It is also antimicrobial and makes a wonderful, moisturizing facemask all by itself. Add it at a 1% dilution to a lotion or lip balm.

Hydrosols

Hydrosols are the water left over after making a steam distillation of an essential oil. They are gentle and tonifying to the skin. They make an excellent ingredient for lotions, creams and toners, or can be used by themselves as a spray directly on the skin. For dry or mature skin: use lavender or rose. Oily or blemished skin is best suited to orange, witch hazel and rosemary. Hydrosols are best stored in dark glass bottles. Store extra in the refrigerator for a longer shelf life. They have a shelf life of 6 months to two years depending on the hydrosol.

Milk

Milk comes from many sources such as cow, goat, sheep, buttermilk, coconut, almond, rice and hemp. Goat's milk has the closest pH to our skin. They are all high in oils and vitamins. Always use full fat, whole, organic milk. I like raw milk the best as it provides more nutrients and enzymes than pasteurized milk. The lactic acid in milk helps exfoliate dead skin cells. It can be used as a facemask, toner, in the bath or as a foot soak in either liquid or powder form. Milk is said to help lighten dark spots on skin. It soothes irritations and smooths and softens the skin.

Oats (*Avena sativa*)

Oats are antioxidant and soothing for rashes, acne and skin irritations. They are hydrating to the skin and make a wonderful addition to a bath or lotion. When ground, rolled oats can be used as a gentle exfoliant or dry shampoo. The anti-inflammatory properties of oats make them soothing for poison ivy, chicken pox, sunburn and eczema. Oats are also used in scrubs, cleansers, soaps and masks.

Sugar cane (*Saccharum officinarum*) or sugar beets (*Beta vulgaris*)

Sugar is a humectant, drawing moisture to and helping to hydrate the skin. It is valuable for both chemical and mechanical exfoliation. Chemically, sugar contains glycolic acid, which helps to break down dead skin cells and clean the pores. Sugar granules are smaller and gentler than salt. For this reason, they are less likely to cause microscopic tears in the skin when used as a scrub. Brown sugar is softer than white sugar. To get even gentler results, you can use powdered brown or white sugar.

Tapioca starch (*Manihot esculenta*)

Derived from the root of the plant, tapioca gives a smooth feeling to the skin and can help control excessive moisture as a body powder or mineral makeup ingredient. It helps keep the skin soft and supple. It is an excellent substitute for cornstarch and is a generally a low allergenic ingredient. Tapioca starch powder is round and smooth, unlike the jagged edges of cornstarch molecules. This makes it gentler for applying on the skin. It can be used in a dilution of 1–15% of a lotion or cream recipe to reduce the oily feeling and increase glide.

Vegetable glycerin

Also called glycerol, vegetable glycerin is a clear, odorless liquid produced from plant oils, typically soy, coconut or palm oil. Avoid glycerin manufactured from animals and synthetic glycerins made from petroleum products as they have less desirable properties. As a humectant, vegetable glycerin draws moisture to the skin. It helps to blend other ingredients together. It softens and soothes skin and is useful for atopic dermatitis, rashes and eczema. It helps oxygenate the skin, provides a protective barrier and encourages healthy skin function. It is used in cosmetics, shampoos, soaps and lotions. Vegetable glycerin has a sweet flavor to it, and is used as an ingredient in lip balms, toothpaste and herbal remedies.

Vitamin C

Vitamin C is a vital nutrient for the skin. It is essential for collagen synthesis, helping to rejuvenate the skin and maintain elasticity. It aids skin healing and is antioxidant, helping to protect against premature aging and cellular damage, particularly UV damage. Vitamin C is available both in water-soluble forms as ascorbic acid or L-ascorbic acid. The fat-soluble form of vitamin C is ascorbyl palmitate, also known as vitamin C ester. A 2002 study by the Mayo Clinic published by the Journal of Investigative Dermatology suggests that although ascorbyl palmitate is more stable in body care products, it is unstable when exposed to the sun and can actually cause massive free radical damage. I suggest avoiding ascorbyl palmitate use in body care products. Ascorbic acid is better absorbed through the skin and although it is less stable, making it difficult to work with, it is far safer. It is likely that including other antioxidants, such as certain herbs and vitamin E, will enhance the stability and shelf life of ascorbic acid. I think the best way to use vitamin C on the skin is to add the fresh powder to water, lotion or cream each morning before applying it, starting with a low dilution of around 5%. If redness or irritation occurs, lower the amount used in your formula. Typically, the amount used would be between 5–20% of a formula.

Yogurt

Yogurt is nourishing and softening to the skin and makes a moisturizing facemask. It can help to improve the skin's microbial balance and help to reduce fungal infections. I find it to be an extremely useful, and simple facemask for acne, aging skin, or dark spots. Just moisten the skin, apply the yogurt over the face and neck, let it sit for 20 minutes, and rinse. The lactic acid in yogurt will helps to dissolve dead skin and tighten pores. Be sure to use live culture, organic, plain, whole fat yogurt.

Natural Preservatives

Natural products will usually have a shorter shelf life than store bought products. Natural preservatives will help extend the shelf life of your body care products. Generally, it is good to make small batches and use them over the span of a few weeks to several months, depending on the product.

There are several things you can do to help your skin care products last longer, slow oxidation and prevent mold and other contaminants from growing. This is especially important for products that contain fixed oils or a combination of oils and waters, such as you would find in a lotion. Most natural products are best kept in a cool, dark location such as the refrigerator.

> *Oil-soluble preservatives are usually antioxidants and will help slow the oxidation process, which causes rancidity in oils. Water-soluble preservatives usually prevent microbial growth in a recipe.*

Some preservatives are water-soluble while others should be added to the oils in your recipe before combining them with the rest of your ingredients. Interestingly, oil-soluble preservatives are usually antioxidants and will help to slow the oxidation process, which causes rancidity in oils. Water-soluble preservatives usually prevent microbial growth in a recipe. Microbial growth is usually only a problem when an ingredient that contains water is used in a recipe. Preservatives are often used as a very small portion of any recipe.

Antioxidant herbs

Many herbs have antioxidant properties that will help preserve your product as well as being beneficial to the skin. The can be added as teas in place of the water portion of a formula, or can be added in small amounts as alcohol extracts (tinctures). A few of my favorite antioxidant herbs for the skin include bilberry or blueberry, cacao, cinnamon, cranberry, sage, green tea, lavender, oregano, pomegranate, rooibos, rose hips, rosemary, thyme, and witch hazel.

Citric acid

Derived from an acid found in many citrus fruits, citric acid is usually obtained in a fermentation process with the bacteria *Aspergillus niger* combined with beet or corn sugar. It works extremely well as a natural preservative by increasing the acidity of a product thereby inhibiting bacteria and mold. It is water and alcohol soluble and can be dissolved in boiled water at the beginning of making your recipe. It can be combined with potassium sorbate to enhance the effectiveness of both. Caution: It can be derived from GMOs. It may irritate sensitive skin. It should be used at 0.3% dilution in your formula.

Essential oils

Essential oils can help to preserve body care products. Although most oils have some antibacterial properties, some of the best antimicrobial oils include caraway, cinnamon, clove, cumin, eucalyptus, lavender, lemon, rose, rosemary, sage, sandalwood and thyme. They are generally used at a 2-10% dilution.

Potassium sorbate

Potassium sorbate is the potassium salt of sorbic acid. Although naturally occurring in some berries, it is almost exclusively manufactured synthetically. It is edible and highly soluble in water. It will help to inhibit microbes such as molds and yeasts. Dissolve it in warm water (70° F or 20° C) when you begin mixing your recipe. It should be used at a .3% dilution.

Rosemary antioxidant

CO_2 is one way used to extract the medicinal properties of plants. Rosemary antioxidant is the CO_2 extraction of the rosemary plant. This oil is useful to preserve fixed oils and butters. It can be used for creams, lotions, body butters, lotion bars and other herbal recipes. The key compound in Rosemary that makes it stabilizing in natural body care products is rosmarinic acid. Rosmarinic acid is a plant-based compound found in a wide variety of spices, but most well known for being an active ingredient in rosemary. It has antioxidant, anti-inflammatory and antimicrobial properties. Add it to the oil part of your mixture. Use it at a .2-.5% dilution.

Vitamin E
Natural vitamin E is derived from soybeans, palm oil, sunflower seeds, wheat germ and other vegetable oils. A powerful antioxidant, vitamin E will help extend the shelf life of fixed oils, lotions, lip balms and salves. Make sure you use natural vitamin E oil (d-alpha tocopherol) as opposed to a synthetic one (labeled with a dl-alpha tocopherol), which is derived from petroleum. Make sure you are getting a non-GMO source. Add it to a fixed oil at 0.5% dilution.

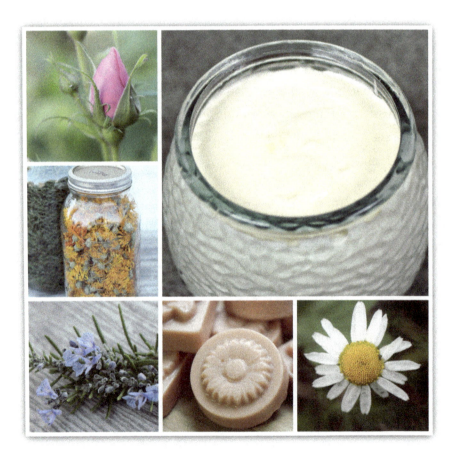

Preservation Suggestions

Because natural body care products don't contain synthetic preservatives, they tend to be more fragile, grow mold and bacteria more easily, and have a shorter shelf life. Along with using natural preservatives, here are some simple practices you can do to help your products last longer.

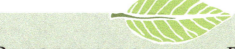

Preserving your Products

- Make sure you are always using the freshest ingredients. It is best to use your raw ingredients within 3 months. Lotions have the shortest shelf life of around one to three months while other body care products can last a year or more.

- Use small containers and keep the bulk of your recipes in the refrigerator. This is mostly important for recipes that contain liquids, especially emulsions such as lotions. Dry products including salts and clays need no special care and are fine stored in a glass jar with a tight fitting lid to reduce water absorption.

- Make sure to wash your hands before making or using products.

- Dispense your lotions and other products with a small spoon or clean chopstick, not your finger. Pump, squeeze and spray bottles also work well, depending on the consistency of your product.

- Make sure all of your bottles, jars, and body care making tools are clean and sterilized before use. Scrubbing well with hot soapy water will get you most of the way there, but they do need to be sterilized by running them through the dishwasher, boiling them, or spraying with full strength vinegar or 25% bleach (my least favorite method) before rinsing. It is also important to make sure each container is airtight to prevent oxidation or exposure to microorganisms.

- Use dark colored, glass containers to reduce oxidation and exposure to light. Glass is also more stable than plastic and will not impart any harmful contaminants into your products.

- If your product has water-based ingredients, always wait until it has cooled before capping, to prevent condensation.

- Make small batches if you will not be using your product quickly.

Skin Types

There are several general skin types that can be helpful to think about when choosing products for the skin. Skin types include mature, oily, normal, dry, problem, sensitive, or a combination of the above. A few skin problems include rosacea, eczema, psoriasis, and acne. Some people have very sensitive and reactive skin. In the following charts, I list general suggestions for several skin types including herbs, clays, natural colorants, essential oils, hydrosols, fixed oils, butters, and other natural ingredients that are beneficial to each skin type.

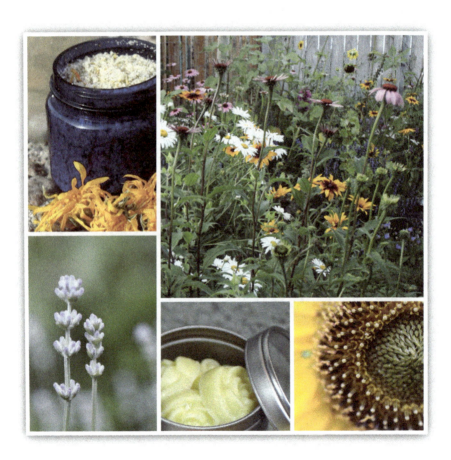

Normal Skin

Normal skin is skin that is functioning properly as an organ. It protects itself well with its natural skin barrier. The skin barrier is a combination of our outer layer of skin, called the epidermis, and the natural oils our skin produces to protect itself. The skin barrier keeps water and vital nutrients in the body as well as keeping microorganisms and damaging substances out of the body.

The skin is intact and the complexion is clear. The other eliminatory organs are working well so the skin does not have to take on extra work. The skin looks healthy and vibrant. People with normal skin can have the occasional breakout or skin issue, but in general the skin is balanced. This type of skin is generally very responsive to most natural body care ingredients.

Skin Care Solutions for Normal Skin	
Herbs	Aloe Vera, Calendula, Chamomile, Chickweed, Comfrey, Elder Flower, Fennel, Green Tea, Lavender, Plantain, Pomegranate, Rooibos, Rose, Rose Hips, Rosemary, Self-Heal, Violet, Witch Hazel, Yarrow
Clays	Bentonite, Kaolin
Natural Colorants	Beet, Cacao, Chlorophyll, Cranberry
Essential Oils	Geranium, Jasmine, Lavender, Neroli, Rose, Thyme linalool, Rosemary
Hydrosols	Chamomile (Roman and German), Lavender, Rose, Rosemary, Witch Hazel
Fixed Oils	Almond, Jojoba, Olive, Walnut
Butters	Carnauba, Cocoa, Coconut, Cupuacu, Kokum, Mango, Shea
Other Natural Ingredients	Honey, Milk, Oats, Vegetable Glycerin, Vitamin C, Yogurt

Oily or Problem Skin

Sometimes the skin gets out of balance. This can be due to stress, hormonal shifts, or diet. The skin tends to mirror our diet and lifestyle. The skin is our largest eliminatory organ and when the other eliminatory organs such as the liver, digestive system, kidneys, or lymph are not working at full capacity, the skin can take on a heavier load.

Topically, make sure you are not stripping the skin of its natural oils, as this will cause excessive oil production as the skin tries harder to balance and protect itself. Use gentle products on the skin to avoid irritation and inflammation. Make sure there is a good microbial balance on the skin. I like to think of it as supporting the skin's ecosystem and cultivating a healthy skin "environment." Avoiding antimicrobial products, both internally and externally, is crucial. Topically, use light oils, yogurt masks, and natural remedies such as healing, anti-inflammatory and antimicrobial herbs and essential oils.

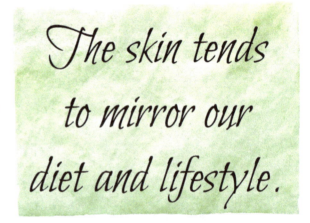

Please be aware when starting to use more natural, healing products, that oily or acne prone skin can sometimes have a cleansing process where things get a little worse before they get better. This is especially true if you have used harsh chemicals or pharmaceuticals on your skin. If your skin is the organ that lets you know when things aren't working well in your body, here is a list of natural remedies you might try. Not all remedies on this list will work well for every person, so experiment and see what works best for your skin.

Skin Care Solutions for Oily or Problem Skin

Herbs	Aloe Vera, Agrimony, Bayberry, Calendula, Cinnamon, Elder Flowers, Geranium, Lavender, Licorice, Oregano, Rooibos, Rose, Rosemary, Sage, Self-Heal, Thyme, Witch Hazel, Yarrow
Clays	Bentonite, Fuller's earth, Kaolin, Red
Natural Colorants	Annatto, Beet, Cacao, Chlorophyll, Cranberry, Turmeric
Essential Oils	Bergapten-free Bergamot*, Cedar, Chamomile (Roman and German), Clary Sage, Cypress, Eucalyptus, Geranium, Juniper, Lavender, Lemongrass, Lemon, Lemon Eucalyptus, Orange, Palmarosa, Rosemary, Sage, Sandalwood, Tea Tree, Thyme
Hydrosols	Frankincense, Lavender, Lemon Balm (Melissa), Lemon Verbena, Orange Flower, Rose, Rosemary, Witch Hazel, Yarrow
Fixed Oils	Avocado, Grape Seed, Hazelnut, Jojoba, Neem, Rosehip Seed, Sea Buckthorn, Walnut
Butters	Kokum, Shea
Other Natural Ingredients	Apple Cider Vinegar, Honey, Lemon Juice, Milk, Oats, Yogurt, Vitamin C

* Bergapten-free Bergamot is an essential oil of bergamot in which the constituent bergapten, which causes photosensitivity, has been removed.

DRY OR SENSITIVE SKIN

Because our skin is our first layer of defense against the outside world, it is important to keep it nourished and hydrated. For those with dry, sensitive, or reactive skin, this can take regular maintenance. It is a good idea to hydrate the skin regularly using gentle hydrosols, emollient herbs, and moisturizing oils and butters.

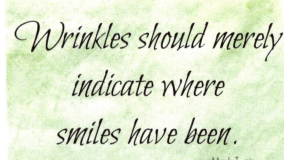

Even so, the skin can react to some recommended ingredients. Try products on the inner elbow before putting them on the face. If redness occurs, avoid that product. If you find yourself having a reaction, discontinue use and keep a note of the ingredients in the recipe you reacted to. This may help you narrow things down to a specific irritant.

Skin Care Solutions for Dry or Sensitive Skin

Herbs	Aloe Vera, Bilberry, Calendula, Chamomile, Chickweed, Cleavers, Comfrey, Elder Flower, Fenugreek, Green Tea, Horsetail, Pomegranate, Kelp, Lavender, Licorice, Marshmallow, Mullein, Plantain, Rose, Violet
Clays	Bentonite, Green, Kaolin
Natural Colorants	Alkanet, Beet, Cacao, Cranberry
Essential Oils	Benzoin, Carrot Seed, Chamomile (Roman and German), Geranium, Lavender, Helichrysum, Jasmine, Neroli, Myrrh, Palmarosa, Patchouli, Rose, Sandalwood, Spikenard, Vetiver, Yarrow, Ylang-ylang
Hydrosols	German Chamomile, Clary Sage, Geranium, Helichrysum, Lavender, Lemon Balm (Melissa), Mrytle, Orange Flower, Rose
Fixed Oils	Almond, Argan, Avocado, Brazil Nut, Cupuacu, Evening Primrose, Hazelnut, Jojoba, Macadamia Nut, Olive, Rosehip Seed, Sea Buckthorn, Sesame
Butters	Carnauba, Cocoa, Coconut, Cupuacu, Kokum, Mango, Shea
Natural Thickeners	Arrowroot, Xanthan Gum
Other Natural Ingredients	Honey, Oats, Milk, Vegetable Glycerin, Vitamin C, Yogurt

Mature Skin

As our skin gets older, it gets thinner and less resilient. We can think of our face as a map of our life, with all the wrinkles, creases, scars, and smile lines mirroring the amazing journey we have had, filled with wisdom, pain, and joy. Antioxidant herbs, vitamin C, and specific butters and fixed oils can be helpful for keeping mature skin moisturized and supple.

Skin Care Solutions for Mature Skin	
Herbs	Aloe Vera, Calendula, Chamomile, Chickweed, Comfrey, Elder Flower, Fennel, Fenugreek, Gotu Kola, Green Tea, Kelp, Lavender, Plantain, Rooibos, Rose, Rose Hips, Self-heal, Violet, Witch Hazel
Clays	Bentonite, Green, Kaolin
Natural Colorants	Beet, Cacao, Chlorophyll, Cranberry
Essential Oils	Carrot Seed, Cistus, Clary Sage, Fennel, Frankincense, Geranium, Helichrysum, Jasmine, Lavender, Myrrh, Myrtle, Neroli, Palmarosa, Patchouli, Rose, Rosemary, Sandalwood, Spikenard
Hydrosols	Carrot Seed, Clary Sage, Geranium, Helichrysum, Lavender, Orange Flower, Rose, Rosemary, Witch Hazel, Yarrow
Fixed Oils	Avocado, Borage, Evening Primrose, Jojoba, Hazelnut, Macadamia Nut, Olive, Rosehip Seed, Sea Buckthorn, Walnut
Butters	Cocoa, Coconut, Cupuacu, Kokum, Mango, Shea
Other Natural Ingredients	Blueberry, Honey, Milk, Vegetable Glycerin, Vitamin C, Yogurt

Recipes for the Body

Caring for our bodies is healing in and of itself. In this age of commercialism, advertising, and airbrushing, it is easy to lose track of the fact that each of our bodies is an amazing and magnificent gift. The mere fact that we have life, that we breathe, move, think, and experience physical sensations is incredible. Every time I think about how the body's many organs and cells work together I am literally awed by the complex synergy of living systems of which we are made. The human body, EVERY human body, is beautiful and astounding to behold.

Taking care of our bodies, by exercising, drinking enough water, eating good food and getting enough sleep are some of the ways we can celebrate our lives and enjoy our physical forms for the miracles they are. Using good and healthy ingredients on our bodies is another way to honor our physicality.

> *Ultimately, it isn't about how we look to the world. What really matters is how we experience this life in our own skin.*

When we take the time and intention to make and use natural body care recipes, we can think of it as helping to keep ourselves healthy and respecting and honoring our bodies. Every time we apply these recipes, we might send a little gratitude to our skin for protecting us so well, or our legs for moving us from place to place, or our eyes for seeing the beauty around us. Ultimately, it isn't about how we look to the world. What really matters is how we experience this life in our own skin.

Herbal Oils

Herbal oils can be used by themselves as a massage oil or for other healing purposes. They can be used as an ingredient in other products such as salves, lotions, ointments, hair oil, lip balms, suppositories, creams, and the list goes on! It is helpful to make some herbal oils to have on hand for your natural body care recipes.

I recommend making herbal oils out of dried herbs whenever possible to lessen the chance of mold or bacterial growth. Most herbs, in my opinion, are best used dry. Some examples are calendula, comfrey, lavender, sage, chamomile, Oregon grape leaf, chaparral, yarrow, witch hazel, cayenne, echinacea, self-heal, plantain, and mullein leaf.

There are only a few herbs I would recommend using fresh, due to their fragile nature. These include arnica, St. John's wort, garlic, and chickweed.

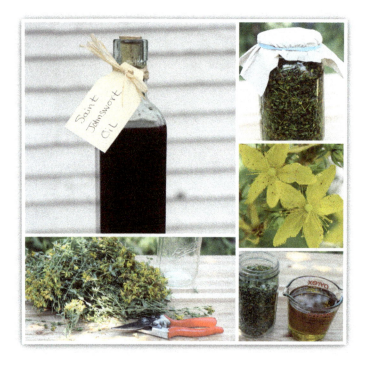

Ingredients:

- Olive oil
- Vitamin E oil
- Benzoin gum
- Essential oils (if desired)
- Herb of your choice

You Will Need:

- Scale
- Measuring cup
- Measuring spoons
- Blender or food processor for dry plants
- Snips or knife for fresh herbs
- Jar with tight-fitting lid (for dry herbs), or muslin cloth or paper towel (for fresh herbs)
- Crock pot, oven or black construction paper if desired
- Strainer
- Bowl
- Herb Press (optional for dry plant oils)

Directions to Make a Dry Plant Oil:

1. Use 1 part dried herb by weight to 7 parts oil by volume. An example would be 2 ounces of echinacea flowers and 14 ounces of olive oil. I like to use extra virgin olive oil as it has its own healing properties for the skin and will infuse well with herbs.
2. Blend the herbs and oil in a blender or food processor until the oil just starts to get warm. This helps the herb infuse into the oil. Some people prefer to heat their oils at a very low temperature in a slow

cooker or the oven. I don't like setting my oils in the sun, as light and heat oxidize oils and they go rancid quicker. To remedy this, you can wrap your jar in black paper before setting it in the sun.

3. You can help your oil infuse by shaking or stirring it once a day.
4. Let your oil infuse for one month.
5. Once it is ready, put a strainer in a bowl and line it with muslin cloth. Pour your oil through the cloth and let it strain. To get any excess, squeeze the herb by hand or press it out with an herb press. Compost your spent herb.
6. To preserve your oil, you can add benzoin gum (1/2 ounce by weight of the powdered gum for every 32 fluid ounces of oil). You can also add Vitamin E oil (1 teaspoon natural vitamin E oil for every 32 fluid ounces of oil). Essential oils will also help preserve your herbal oils and provide their own healing properties. Add 10–12 drops per ounce of oil.
7. Dry plant oils have a shelf life of 1–2 years. Store your oil in a glass jar in a cool, dark place such as the refrigerator or a cupboard.

Directions to Make a Fresh Plant Oil:

1. Wilt herbs in a dark, cool place (paper bag or screen) for several hours or overnight to reduce their water content.
2. Use 1 part herb by weight to 4 parts oil by volume. An example of this would be 2 ounces of garlic to 8 ounces of olive oil.
3. Chop the herb well before adding the oil. Do not grind it.
4. Make sure the herb is completely covered in oil. Parts that stick out will tend to mold.
5. Cover the jar with a paper towel or cheesecloth to allow moisture from the herbs to evaporate. This is a crucial step to prevent mold. I have even heard of jars exploding when this step is not followed.
6. Infuse for 1 month in cool dark place. St. John's wort needs to be warmed, which can be done by putting it in the sun (I like to wrap black construction paper around the jar first to protect it from the

light), or baked in an oven or cooked in a crockpot for 2 hours on the lowest heat.
7. Once it is ready, put a strainer in a bowl and line it with muslin cloth. Pour your oil through the cloth and let it strain.
8. To avoid getting moisture from the plant into the oil, squeeze fresh plant oils out by hand through a muslin cloth or cheesecloth. If you do get water into your oil, decant as needed to remove it. Water will sink to the bottom of the jar and not incorporate with the oil. It can cause mold.
9. To preserve your oil, you can add benzoin gum (1/2 ounce by weight of the powdered gum for every 32 fluid ounces of oil). You can also add vitamin E oil (1 teaspoon natural vitamin E oil for every 32 fluid ounces of oil). Essential oils will also help preserve your herbal oils and provide their own healing properties. Add 10–12 drops per ounce of oil.
10. Fresh plant oils have a shelf life of up to one year or more. They are best refrigerated.

ALOE VERA GEL

Aloe vera gel is soothing and moisturizing to the skin. It is an excellent remedy to have on hand for dry skin, burns, scrapes, abrasions, pimples, bites, and stings, and to soothe sunburn.

You don't have to purchase aloe gel from the store to use this plant. Caution must be used, however, when making your own gel as aloe latex (yellow in color), which is just below the outer leaf surface, is a very potent and uncomfortable laxative when ingested.

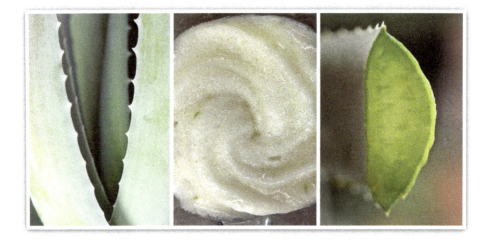

Homemade aloe gel can be used by itself or added to a body care recipe. As it has not been over processed, it has all of its fresh healing properties intact. It is much thicker and more mucilaginous than the store bought variety and will have a shorter shelf life. It can make your recipe thicker and slightly more unpredictable than using a store bought gel in your recipe. Here is the recipe to make your own aloe vera gel.

Ingredients:

- Measure by volume:
    - ½ cup aloe vera gel (you will need 2–3 large fronds for this)
    - ¼ teaspoon citric acid
    - 20–40 drops of essential oil if desired (essential oils will help to prolong the shelf life of this recipe)

You Will Need:

- Healthy aloe vera plant
- Sharp knife
- Vegetable/fruit peeler
- Spoon or butter knife
- Measuring cup
- Measuring spoon
- Bowl
- Blender or Cuisinart

Directions:

1. To harvest aloe, choose a healthy leaf from the base of a plant. Cut close to the main stem, using a sharp knife.
2. Let the leaf sit upside down in a cup or bowl for 10–15 minutes to let the yellow latex drain out.
3. Carefully remove the outer skin (rind) of the leaf with a sharp knife or a vegetable/fruit peeler. The gel can be scooped out of the outer skin with a spoon or butter knife into a bowl.
4. Any residual yellow latex should be washed off the inner gel.
5. Add all ingredients together and blend.
6. This gel has a shelf life of several months when stored in the refrigerator.

Healing Garden Salve

This is a wonderful all-purpose salve for healing the skin. It can be used for scrapes, cuts, stings, abrasions, skin irritations, cracks, diaper rash, and rough cuticles. It is also useful for mild infections and inflammations of the skin. Do not use on deep wounds, as salves should not be applied deep into the body tissues. Once a wound has healed from the inside, salves can be applied to reduce scarring and speed the final healing process.

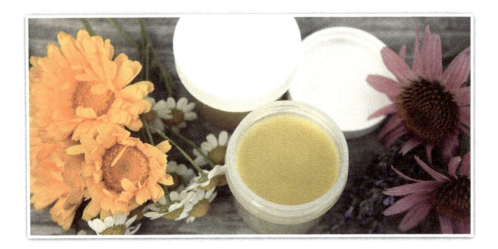

Ingredients:

- Measure by volume:
    - 2 ounces self-heal oil
    - 2 ounces plantain oil
    - 2 ounces calendula oil
    - 2 ounces comfrey oil
    - 2 ounces echinacea root or flower oil
    - 60 drops lavender essential oil
    - 20 drops Roman chamomile essential oil
- Measure by weight:
    - 2 1/2 ounces beeswax

You Will Need:
- Scale
- Measuring cup
- Double boiler
- Spoon
- Small plate
- Salve jars or large lip balm tubes (these work nicely for applying salves)
- Labels

Directions:
1. Firstly, make or purchase your herbal oils (see Herbal Oils). I like to make each oil separately so I can use them by themselves, or have the opportunity to mix them in other recipes later. Alternately, you can throw them all together and make a combined oil.
2. Add equal parts of each oil together and set aside.
3. You will need 25% beeswax, by weight, to make your oils into a salve. For example, if you have 4 ounces of herbal oil, use 1 ounce of beeswax. You can use a bit less beeswax if you prefer a softer salve, or a bit more beeswax if you like your salve harder.
4. Melt your beeswax in double boiler until it is liquid. There is no need to grate it first.
5. Add the herbal oils.
6. Stir well until beeswax and oil are incorporated and completely melted.
7. You can also add other oils or butters such as lanolin, cocoa butter or coconut oil for a more creamy consistency. It is fun to experiment with your own recipes!
8. You can check for consistency with a spoon and plate. Just spoon a little salve onto your plate and let it cool. It is easy to adjust your consistency by adding more oil or beeswax at this point.
9. Remove your pan from heat and add essential oils if desired.
10. Pour into containers cap and label.

Deep Muscle Salve

This deep muscle rub can be used for bruises, injuries, joint pain, arthritis and sore or overworked muscles. Use Deep Muscle Salve before working out to warm the muscles and after exercise to speed recovery. Do not use this salve on broken skin as it can cause irritation.

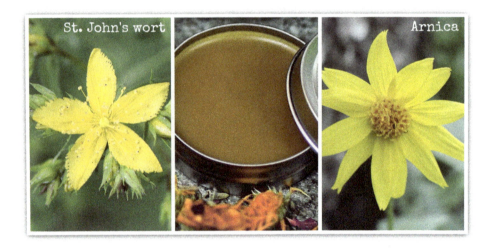

Ingredients:

- Measure by volume:
    - 2 ounces St. John's wort oil
    - 2 ounces arnica oil
    - 2 ounce poplar oil
    - 30 drops birch essential oil
    - 30 drops camphor essential oil
    - 20 drops cinnamon essential oil
    - 20 drops ginger essential oil
    - 4 drops clove essential oil
- Measure by weight
    - 1.5 ounces beeswax

You Will Need:

- Scale
- Measuring cup
- Double boiler
- Spoon
- Small plate
- Salve jars or large lip balm tubes (these work nice for applying salves)
- Labels

Directions:

1. Firstly, make or purchase your herbal oils (see Herbal Oils). I like to make each oil separately so I can use them by themselves, or have the opportunity to mix them in other recipes later. Alternately, you can throw them all together and make a combined oil.
2. Add 2 ounces of each oil together and set aside.
3. Melt your beeswax in double boiler until it is liquid. There is no need to grate it first.
4. Add the herbal oils.
5. Stir well until beeswax and oil are incorporated and completely melted.
6. You can also add other oils or butters such as mango butter, kokum butter, cocoa butter or coconut oil for a more creamy consistency. Have fun getting creative and designing your own recipes!
7. You can check for consistency with a spoon and plate. Just spoon a little salve onto your plate and let it cool. It is easy to adjust your consistency by adding more oil or beeswax at this point.
8. Remove your pan from heat and add essential oils if desired.
9. Pour into containers cap and label.

Green Biotic Ointment

This recipe is similar to a salve, but softer, making it easier to apply to painful or infected areas. Green Biotic Ointment is useful for cuts, scrapes, infections, and hot, irritated skin. It has a high percentage of essential oils to increase its antimicrobial and antifungal properties. For children or those with sensitive skin, you can reduce the amount of essential oils if desired. I recommend keeping some Green Biotic Ointment in your medicine cabinet as well as in your first aid kit.

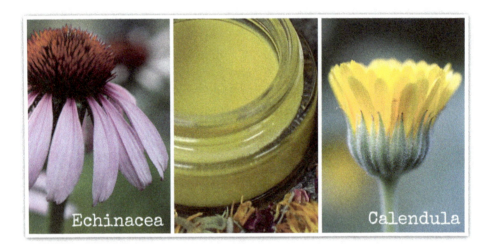

Ingredients:

- Measure by volume:
    - 2 ounces calendula oil
    - 2 ounce echinacea flower (or root) oil
    - ½ teaspoon vitamin E oil
    - 60 drops tea tree essential oil
    - 60 drops thyme linalool essential oil
    - 30 drops cinnamon essential oil
    - 30 drops oregano essential oil

- Measure by weight:
    - 2 ounces shea butter
    - 2 ounces coconut oil
    - 1 ounce kokum butter
    - .5 ounce beeswax

You Will Need:

- Double boiler
- Thermometer
- Measuring cup
- Scale
- Measuring spoons
- Salve jars
- Labels

Directions:

1. To prevent graininess, heat the kokum and shea butters to 150°F (65° C) in the double boiler if desired.
2. Add the beeswax and coconut oil and let melt, stirring well.
3. Add the herbal oils and let heat until just melted, stirring well.
4. Remove from the heat and add the essential oils.
5. Pour into jars, cap, and label.

Aromatic Chest Rub

The Aromatic Chest Rub is useful for coughs, congestion, colds, respiratory infections, and bronchitis. This balm can be rubbed on the chest, back, and neck. This formula has a high percentage of essential oils. If desired, you can reduce the drops for those with sensitive skin and small children.

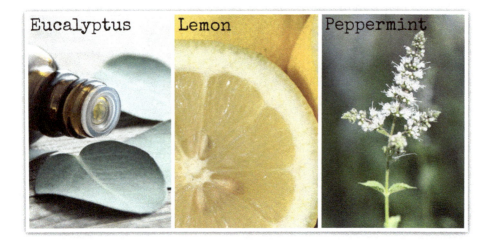

Ingredients:

- Measure by volume:
    - 4 ounces almond oil
    - ½ teaspoon vitamin E oil
    - 20 drops *Eucalyptus radiata* essential oil
    - 20 drops thyme linalool essential oil
    - 20 drops pine essential oil
    - 20 drops lemon essential oil
    - 20 drops peppermint essential oil
    - 20 drops cypress essential oil

- Measure by weight:
    - 2 ounces shea butter
    - 2 ounces coconut oil
    - 1 ounce kokum butter
    - .5 ounce beeswax

You Will Need:

- Double boiler
- Thermometer
- Measuring cup
- Scale
- Measuring spoons
- Salve jars
- Labels

Directions:

6. To prevent graininess, heat the kokum and shea butters to 150°F (65° C) in the double boiler if desired.
7. Add the beeswax and coconut oil and let melt, stirring well.
8. Add the almond oil and let heat until just melted, stirring well.
9. Remove from the heat and add the essential oils.
10. Pour into jars, cap and label.

Moisturizing Lotion Bar

This is a solid lotion bar that is handy to use for travel. You can carry a small bar in a purse or backpack. I like to have a bar handy by my kitchen and bathroom sinks. It is especially hydrating to use a bar after a bath or shower. You can vary the ingredients to make bars specific for the face, hardworking hands, cracked feet, pregnant bellies, baby bottoms, and more. You can make smaller-sized bars for travel, to give as gifts, or to carry inside a purse or backpack.

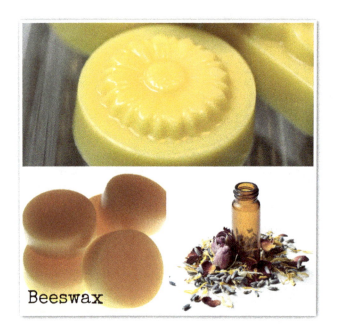

Ingredients:

- Measure by weight:
    - 5 ounces beeswax (you can add less beeswax in the winter if desired for a softer consistency)
    - 7 ounces cocoa butter
    - 4 ounces coconut oil
    - 4 ounces almond oil

- Measure by volume:
    - 1 teaspoon vitamin E oil
    - 1 teaspoon essential oil of your choice. I like lavender, geranium, rosemary, or lemongrass.

You Will Need:

- Scale
- Double boiler
- Metal spoon
- Glass Pyrex measuring cup
- Molds including candy molds, soap molds or even ice cube trays.

Directions:

1. Melt the beeswax in a double boiler.
2. Add the cocoa butter and coconut oil and stir until melted.
3. Add the almond oil and vitamin E oil and stir once again until melted.
4. Add your essential oil(s) and stir well.
5. Wipe off the bottom of the double boiler to remove any excess water.
6. Pour into a Pyrex measuring cup.
7. Pour into molds.
8. Let cool and then pop the bars out of the mold.
9. I like to store bars in small metal tins for portability.

Lotion Bar Variations:

Here are some additional ingredients you can add to your lotion bars to make them more specific for various skin care applications.

Sunscreen or Diaper Rash Bar

- Add 1 cup zinc oxide or titanium dioxide. This will give you an SPF of approximately 25. Make sure you run your oxide through a strainer, flour sifter or powder it with a mortar and pestle to break up any clumps before using. When working with clays, it is good to wear a mask or bandana over the nose and mouth.

Exfoliating Bar

- Add ground lavender, oatmeal, or dried coffee grounds.

Bug Repellant Bar

- 60 drops lavender essential oil
- 60 drops lemongrass essential oil
- 30 drops red thyme essential oil
- 30 drops lemon essential oil
- 30 drops peppermint essential oil

Deodorant Bar

- ½ cup arrowroot powder
- 1 tablespoon baking soda
- 2 teaspoons lavender, tea tree or cedar essential oil

- You can use this under your arms or on your feet.

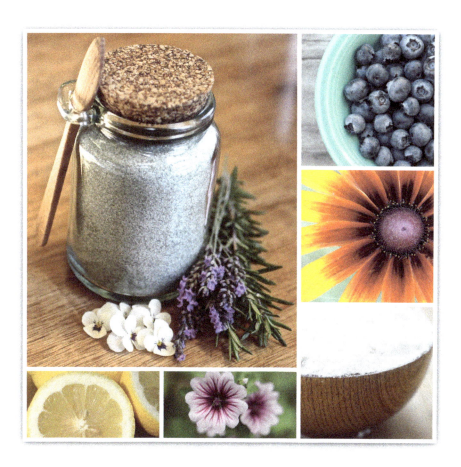

Shea Lavender Whipped Body Butter

You can use this delectable butter on your entire body including your face. It is light, fluffy, and soaks in well without leaving an oily residue. Shea Lavender Body Butter makes a lovely and inexpensive gift! This is a large recipe, good for gift giving or sharing with friends. It contains no water so it will have a longer shelf life of a year or so depending on the freshness of your ingredients.

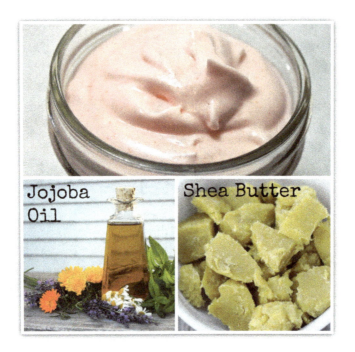

Ingredients:

- Measure by weight:
    - 4 ounces shea butter
    - 1 pound 12 ounces virgin coconut oil
- Measure by volume:
    - 3/4 cup almond oil (you can substitute an herbal oil here)
    - 1/4 cup jojoba oil

- 1 teaspoon vitamin E oil
- 2 tablespoons alkanet root (for a pink color, if desired)
- 50 drops lavender essential oil (or any other essential oils you like)

You Will Need:

- Scale
- Double boiler
- Large bowl
- Strainer
- Blender
- Glass jars
- Labels

Directions:

1. Melt shea butter and coconut oil in a double boiler. Stir well.
2. Once completely melted, remove the pan and pour into a large bowl.
3. Let cool until the oils start solidifying on the sides of the bowl. This step can take several hours, and can be expedited up by putting the bowl in the refrigerator for a while.
4. Meanwhile, add the alkanet root to the almond oil. It infuses very fast and should be ready to strain as your coconut/shea mixture is finishing cooling.
5. Strain the alkanet root from the almond oil. You can compost the spent alkanet root.
6. Add all ingredients together.
7. Blend, blend, and blend. This step can take a while. You can watch your recipe get fluffier as more air is incorporated into the oils.
8. You can put the oil into the refrigerator occasionally to speed this process.

9. Scrape the sides of the bowl every once in a while. It takes a while, but you will end up with a light, creamy butter that is wonderful for the whole body.
10. Put in jars right away, as the mixture will harden as it cools completely.
11. Enjoy!

Tropical Body Butter

Whether in the heat of summer or the dryness of winter, our skin needs loving care to make sure it stays smooth, resilient, and moisturized. Body butters help to seal in the skin's moisture and improve its barrier function, adding softness and health to the largest organ of our body. This recipe can be used daily all over the body, as well as the elbows, knees, heels, hands, and cuticles.

Ingredients:

- Measure by weight:
    - 4 ounces virgin coconut oil
    - 2 ounces shea butter
    - 2 ounces mango butter
- Measure by volume:
    - 1 tablespoon jojoba oil
    - 1 teaspoon castor oil
    - ½ teaspoon vitamin E oil
    - 35 drops bay laurel essential oil
    - 35 drops orange essential oil
    - 14 drops cardamom essential oil
    - 7 drops benzoin essential oil

You Will Need:

- Scale
- Measuring spoons
- Double boiler
- Glass containers
- Labels

Directions:

1. If desired, first temper the shea and mango butters by heating them to 175° F (80° C) in a double boiler. Then cool the butters to about 70° F (21° C).
2. Then add the coconut oil, jojoba oil, vitamin E oil and castor oil, gently warming until they are all melted and thoroughly combined.
3. Allow the mixture to cool for 15 minutes and add the essential oils.
4. Pour into a glass container with a tight-fitting lid.

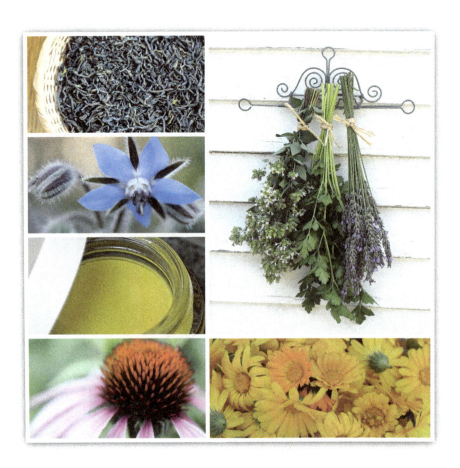

Eczema Balm

Eczema is a condition that causes the skin to become inflamed and irritated. It is a complex health issue that often involves inflammation, food allergies, and sometimes a predisposition to asthma. Along with dealing with the internal causes of eczema such as diet, external skin support is a must. This recipe helps moisturize, reduce inflammation, and soothe itching as well as helping to repair and restore the skin. It is helpful to apply this blend every day. Make sure to apply it after bathing. This recipe can be used on both the face and body. It smells divine!

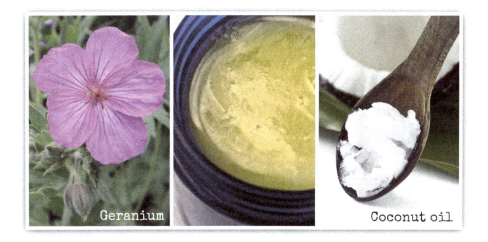
Geranium   Coconut oil

Ingredients:

- Measure by weight
    - 1 ounce beeswax
    - 1 ounce kokum butter
    - 4 ounces coconut oil
- Measure by volume:
    - 5 ounces calendula oil
    - 1 tablespoon evening primrose, borage, or avocado oil
    - ½ teaspoon vitamin E oil or 1 ¼ teaspoon rosemary antioxidant

- 30 drops geranium essential oil
- 30 drops German chamomile essential oil
- 30 drops lavender essential oil
- 30 drops palmarosa essential oil

You Will Need:

- Scale
- Measuring cups and spoons
- Double boiler
- Spatula
- Jars
- Labels

Directions:

1. In a double boiler, melt the beeswax and kokum butter. You can temper the kokum butter by heating to 175° F (80° C) if desired. Then let cool to 70° F (21° C).
2. Add the calendula oil, coconut oil and vitamin E oil to the double boiler and heat until melted. Stir well.
3. Remove from the heat and add your evening primrose, borage, or avocado oil. Mix well.
4. Let cool for 5–15 minutes.
5. Add the essential oils, pour into jars and cap.
6. This recipe can be used on the face and the body.
7. If additional moisture is desired, you can spray the skin with Lavender Face Toner before applying Eczema Balm.

Soothing Sitz Bath

A sitz bath is a bath used for healing purposes, where only the bottom and hips are immersed in the water. Sitz baths help bring blood to the area, which brings more nutrients and helps carry away waste products. This helps the body maintain healthy tissue and helps to heal wounds, infections or resolve stagnant conditions. Sitz baths can be soothing to inflamed or injured tissue. Sitz baths increase lymphatic drainage, which helps eliminate wastes and is crucial for the immune response in the body. They are valuable for both men and women.

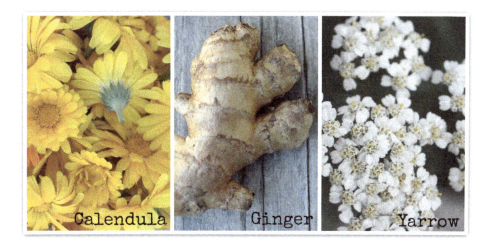

Sitz baths are helpful for supporting the health of the lower abdomen, including the reproductive system and lower GI tract, and especially the rectum and anus. They are useful for reproductive health issues, infections, herpes outbreaks, hemorrhoids, and infertility. Men should avoid hot baths when trying to have a child with their partner. Sitz baths are commonly used after childbirth. For this purpose, use only a warm, not hot, bath and do not use the cold bath. Pregnant women should avoid sitz baths.

Many herbs can be used in a sitz bath for their healing properties such as calendula, chamomile, comfrey, echinacea, geranium, ginger, lavender, licorice, Oregon grape root, plantain, rose, sage, self-heal, uva ursi, witch hazel, and yarrow.

Ingredients:

- ¼ ounce of each of the following herbs, by weight:
    - Calendula
    - Yarrow
    - Ginger
    - Licorice
    - Witch hazel
    - Uva ursi
- 5 cups of water

You Will Need:

- Scale
- Teapot or pot with a lid
- Strainer
- Two large containers that you can sit in. Plastic bins work well or you can buy a special sitz bath container. One "container" can be your bathtub.

Directions:

1. Bring water to a boil and pour over the herbs.
2. Cover and let the tea steep for ½ hour and then strain.
3. Make sure your bathroom or bathing area is warm and comfy.
4. Fill one container with hot water (not too hot, but very warm) and add your herbal tea. Fill the tub full enough so when you sit in it, the water will not come up over your stomach. The idea is to focus the water on the pelvic region. Do not submerge legs, arms, back, or other parts of your body.

5. Fill the other container with very cold water. Fill the tub full enough so when you sit in it, the water will not come up over your stomach.
6. Sit in the warm water for 3 minutes. Then switch to the cold water for 30 seconds. Repeat 3 times, ending with the cold water.
7. You will notice a distinct tingling, the feeling of increased circulation to the area.
8. Sitz baths should be done from 3 to 5 times a week, depending on the health situation and progress of the person.

In order to keep all ingredients fresh, make a new batch of tea each time you do a sitz bath. Alternately, the tea can also be frozen in ice cube trays for later use.

Varicose Vein Refresher

This stimulating blend is wonderful for small spider veins, as well as for refreshing tired arms and legs. It makes an invigorating spray for those who are on their feet for long periods of time.

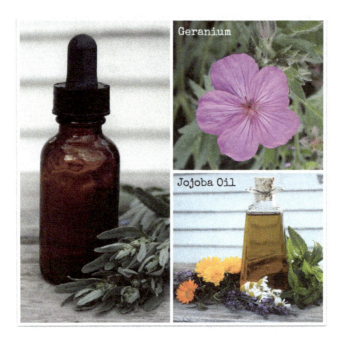

Ingredients:

- Measure by volume:
    - 3 ounces witch hazel extract
    - 1 ounce yarrow tincture
    - 1 teaspoon jojoba oil
    - 20 drops geranium essential oil
    - 15 drops cypress essential oil
    - 10 drops lemon essential oil
    - 5 drops peppermint essential oil

You Will Need:

- Measuring cups
- Measuring spoons
- Bowl or jar
- Glass bottles
- Labels

Directions:

1. Mix all ingredients well.
2. Pour into a dark glass spray or dropper bottle and label.
3. Shake well before applying to legs, arms or wherever you have varicose veins.
4. For extra benefit, put your feet up and relax for 10–20 minutes.

Citrus Almond Body Scrub

This soothing and invigorating scrub offers a gentle way to remove dead skin, encourage circulation, and rid the skin of impurities without being too drying. It makes a valuable treatment for cellulite and to move stagnant lymph. After using Citrus Almond Body Scrub, your skin will feel supple, smooth, and delightfully soft!

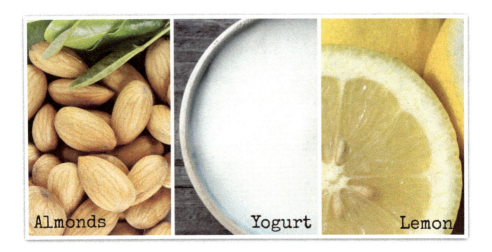

Almonds — Yogurt — Lemon

Ingredients:

- Measure by volume:
    - 2 tablespoons kaolin clay
    - 2 tablespoons almonds
    - 2 tablespoons oats
    - 2 tablespoons finely powdered lemon or orange peel
    - 1/4 cup yogurt
    - Juice of 1 small fresh lemon
    - 1 tablespoon almond oil
    - 40 drops juniper essential oil
    - 20 drops lemon essential oil
    - 20 drops orange essential oil

You Will Need:

- Measuring cups
- Measuring spoons
- Blender or coffee grinder
- Spoon
- Metal bowl
- Strainer for the bathtub. There are different varieties of these ranging from plastic to metal. Cheesecloth can work in a pinch.

Directions:

1. Grind the almonds and oats, making sure they are uniform and a little gritty.
2. Mix with the kaolin clay and powdered citrus peel.
3. At this point, you can make some extra to be stored in a jar for later use if you wish.
4. Add the lemon juice, yogurt, almond oil, and essential oils.
5. Add water as needed to get a consistency that you like.
6. Wet your skin with a brief shower.
7. Sitting naked in an empty bathtub, use a circular motion to gently massage the scrub into the face and skin, moving from the extremities towards the heart. This process is especially helpful for moving the lymph.
8. Sit for 10 minutes and let the mixture dry and pull out any impurities from the skin.
9. Before rinsing, place your strainer for the bathtub over the drain.
10. Shower and enjoy the feeling of soft and radiant skin, naturally!
11. Citrus Almond Body Scrub can be used weekly as an invigorating treatment.

Citrus Body Oil

As a follow up for Citrus Almond Body Scrub, you can apply Citrus Body Oil daily to any areas of cellulite that you would like to focus on. This product is best used in the evening or under clothing. Do not expose the skin to sunlight while wearing Citrus Body Oil as citrus oils are photosensitizing and can cause sunburn.

Ingredients:

- Measure by volume:
    - 1 ounce almond oil
    - 20 drops juniper essential oil
    - 10 drops lemon essential oil
    - 10 drops orange essential oil

You Will Need:

- Measuring cups
- Measuring spoons
- Dark glass container
- Label

Directions:

1. Mix all ingredients together and pour in your dark glass bottle.
2. To use, massage into the skin vigorously.
3. A natural bristle skin brush can be used to stimulate lymph and circulation if desired. Always brush toward the heart.

Sugar and Spice Body Scrub

This simple body scrub helps to exfoliate dead skin cells, stimulate the lymph system, and revitalize the skin. This is a great scrub to use during a morning shower.

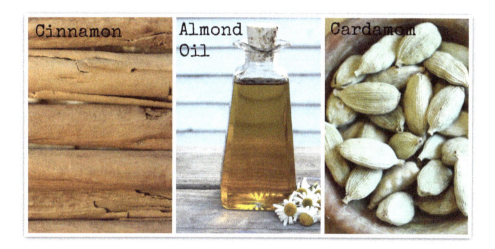

Ingredients:

- Measure by volume:
    - 2 cups brown sugar
    - ¾ cup almond oil
    - ¼ cup jojoba oil
    - 1 teaspoon vitamin E oil
    - 30 drops bergamot essential oil
    - 20 drops benzoin essential oil
    - 15 drops cinnamon essential oil
    - 15 drops cardamom essential oil

You Will Need:

- Large bowl
- Measuring cups

- Measuring spoons
- Spoon
- Glass jar with tight-fitting lid
- Labels

Directions:

1. Mix all ingredients together and store in a jar with a tight-fitting lid. Make sure the jar has a wide mouth so you can get your hand in it.
2. At the end of a relaxing shower or bath, massage the Sugar and Spice Body Scrub into your skin, starting with your feet and working your way towards your heart.
3. Breathe deeply.
4. Shower off and pat gently dry.
5. For a warmer wintertime blend, try these essential oils instead: ginger, cardamom, and orange.

Sparkle Body Powder

Traditionally, body powders are made from a mineral known as talc. Talc can be contaminated with asbestos and studies have shown even asbestos-free talc can cause potential toxicity and problems such as cancer. This recipe is a smooth and effective natural body powder with no talc in it. This blend is cooling and refreshing. Use some Sparkle Body Powder and add a little shimmer to your day!

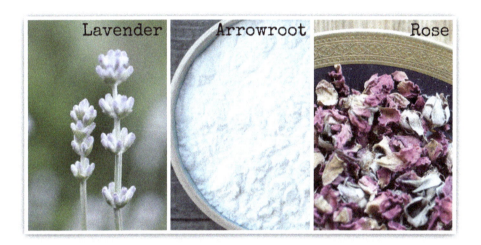

Ingredients:

- Measure by volume:
    - ½ cup kaolin clay
    - 1 cup arrowroot powder or cornstarch
    - 1/8 cup powdered dry rose petals
    - 2 tablespoons powdered mica (optional to add sparkle!)
    - 40 drops tea tree, lavender or peppermint essential oil, depending on your preference

You Will Need:

- Measuring cups
- Measuring spoons
- Large bowl
- Blender or coffee grinder
- Glass jars
- Labels

Directions:

1. Mix all ingredients together.
2. Blend thoroughly if there are any clumps or larger pieces.
3. Store in an airtight glass jar.
4. Use liberally and shimmer like a summer day.

Bug Be Gone Oil

This is a wonderful and versatile aromatherapy blend for keeping those pesky bugs at bay. You can use it on your body or around the area you are in to deter mosquitoes, flies and other biting insects.

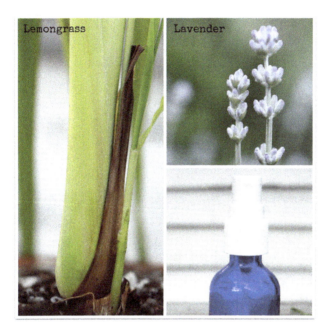

Ingredients:

- 10 drops lavender essential oil
- 8 drops lemongrass essential oil
- 4 drops red thyme essential oil
- 4 drops lemon essential oil
- 4 drops peppermint essential oil
- Optional ingredients, depending on how you want to use this blend, include 2 ounces of the following: fixed oil, vodka, ethyl alcohol, witch hazel, or water

You Will Need:

- Glass spray bottle
- Label
- Measuring cup
- Different items depending on how you choose to use your oil blend. See "How to Use It" below.

Directions:

1. Mix all oils together.
2. Store in a glass bottle.

How to Use It:

- Dab some on a cotton ball and set it near you
- Add 3–10 drops to a candle
- Put several drops on lengths of ribbon and hang them around your room or outside
- Add 30 drops to 2 ounces vegetable oil and use liberally directly on the skin.
- Add 30 drops to 2 ounces water, vodka, witch hazel, or ethyl alcohol (such as Everclear). This recipe can be put in a glass spray bottle and used to spray on the skin, hair, clothes, or surrounding areas. Shake well before use.

Recipes for the Face

Our face is what we present to the world. Humans have 42 individual muscles in their face. We use these muscles to communicate our emotions, thoughts, and inner experiences to the world. It is wonderful when our inner vibrancy and beauty can shine out through our face.

The skin on the face is thinner than the skin on the rest of the body. It is also constantly exposed to the elements, air pollution, and sun, and so needs extra care. I recommend a simple daily face care regimen of cleansing, toning, and moisturizing. Once a week, if desired or needed, you can give some kind of an extra treat to your skin such as a *gentle* exfoliation or facemask. Make sure to treat your scalp, neck, and chest as an extension of your face.

> *If you have good thoughts they will shine out of your face like sunbeams and you will always look lovely.*
> ~ Roald Dahl

Almond Cream Cleanser

This is a gentle and non-stripping cleanser that works great for makeup removal. It will clean the face without stripping the skin's own natural oils. It can even be used as a light moisturizer for the hands or face, or as a serum base by adding additional ingredients such as vitamin C or E, precious essential oils, beta glucans, antioxidant herbs, or small amounts of fixed oils including sea buckthorn, borage, avocado, and rosehip seed oil.

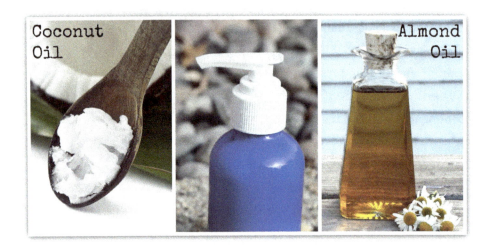

Ingredients:

- Measure by volume:
    - 1/4 teaspoon xanthan gum
    - ½ cup hydrosol (I like lavender)
    - 1/8 teaspoon citric acid
    - 1 tablespoon coconut oil
    - ¼ cup almond oil
    - ½ teaspoon lanolin
    - ¼ teaspoon vitamin E oil
    - ½ teaspoon tea tree essential oil (or other essential oil if desired)
    - 1 teaspoon stearic acid

You Will Need:

- Whisk
- Glass or stainless steel bowl
- Double boiler
- Blender
- Jars
- Labels

Directions:

1. Make sure all utensils, tools, and containers are sterilized before use.
2. Slowly whisk the xanthan gum and citric acid into the hydrosol and let sit for 15 minutes to thicken.
3. Melt coconut oil and stearic acid in a double boiler.
4. Once melted, take off heat, add almond oil, lanolin, and vitamin E oil and stir well.
5. Let the oils cool to room temperature.
6. Once cool, add your essential oil.
7. The two mixtures should be approximately the same temperature to mix properly.
8. Pour the hydrosol mixture into the blender and mix until all the clumps are gone.
9. Turn the blender on high and slowly drizzle the oil mixture into the blender until all ingredients make a creamy, consistent mixture.
10. Pour into jars or bottles. I like to use a glass dropper or pump bottle.
11. Let cool completely before capping.
12. Store any extra in the refrigerator.

Vitamin C Serum

Vitamin C is one of the very best nutrients we can apply to our skin. Prolonged, consistent use of Vitamin C Serum will cause the body to produce more collagen. Collagen is the main structural protein found in the skin and is essential for skin repair after injury. When using this serum, skin will likely look plumper, more moisturized, tighter and less wrinkled. Vitamin C is also valuable for lightening dark spots on the skin and helping to heal acne and scars. Vitamin C is antioxidant, protecting the skin from free-radical damage. It can take 3–6 months to see results of collagen production, although some people report results much sooner.

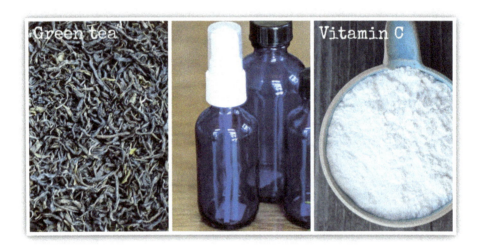

For the serum to be effective, the pH needs to be 3.5–3.0. Make sure it doesn't go below 3.0 as it can be irritating or damaging to the skin. To check acidity, use a pH strip. Vitamin C can cause irritation, so start with a low dilution, such as 5%. Every two weeks, raise your vitamin C content an additional 5% in your serum until you get to between 10–20%. If the serum is stinging or causing redness, lower the dilution. If you have sensitive skin, test on your inner arm before applying to the face. Combining vitamin C with vitamin E (the water soluble form is best for this formula), and antioxidant herbs such as green tea will increase the effectiveness of the serum.

Vitamin C oxidizes quickly so the serum should be made in frequent, small batches. For maximum freshness and bioavailability, make a new batch every three days or so. The serum will tend to last longer with other antioxidants such as green tea and vitamin E. If the serum begins to rise or turn yellow, or the pH rises over 3.5, discard it and make a new batch.

Ingredients:

- Measure by volume:
    - Vitamin C powder (either ascorbic acid or L-ascorbic acid), see amounts on the Vitamin C Serum Solutions Chart below
    - ½ teaspoon vegetable glycerin
    - ¾ teaspoon vitamin E (optional, water soluble is preferable)
    - 1 cup boiling water
- Measure by weight:
    - ¼ ounce green tea leaves

You Will Need:

- Measuring spoons
- Strainer
- Dark glass jars with tight-fitting dropper lid or sprayer
- pH strips
- Label
- Tea pot or canning jar
- Small bowl
- Spoon
- Small funnel

Directions:

1. Make a strong infusion of your green tea by first boiling the water.
2. Pour 1 cup of water over .25 ounce green tea leaves.
3. Let steep 2 hours and strain.

4. Let cool to room temperature before adding other ingredients.
5. You can freeze the excess green tea infusion in ice cube trays for later use.
6. Mix 1 ounce of green tea with vegetable glycerin and vitamin E (if desired) and store in a dark bottle. For simplicity, I call this the "antioxidant base blend." Store this blend in the refrigerator to use as your carrier serum for the vitamin C.
7. You can play with the amount of vegetable glycerin that you prefer. The more glycerin, the more moisturizing the formula is. In excess, glycerin can leave a tacky feeling to the skin.
8. In a smaller bottle (I like to use a dark glass spray bottle), add your exact amounts of the antioxidant base blend and the vitamin C. A small funnel is helpful. Shake well until the vitamin C has dissolved completely.
9. Check your pH to make sure it is 3.5–3.0. If your blend is too acidic (lower than 3.0), add a pinch of baking soda. If it is too alkaline (above 3.5), add a pinch of citric acid.
10. Shake well before applying, as the vitamin E will not dissolve in the formula.
11. Apply this serum at night after cleansing and toning and before you apply a moisturizer. If desired, you can use it all over your body, focusing on problem areas such as dark spots, acne, scars, and the face and hands.
12. Store in a cool dark location such as the medicine cabinet.

Vitamin C Serum Solutions

5% Solution	1 ounce antioxidant base blend
	1/3 teaspoon ascorbic acid
10% Solution	1 ounce antioxidant base blend
	2/3 teaspoon ascorbic acid
15% Solution	1 ounce antioxidant base blend
	1 scant teaspoon ascorbic acid
20% Solution	1 ounce antioxidant base blend
	1 1/4 scant teaspoons ascorbic acid

Lavender Face Toner

This inexpensive, simple recipe is my favorite face toner of all time. It is gentle, hydrating, and nourishing to the skin. I love the way it smells and the way it makes my skin feel.

Ingredients:

- Measure by volume:
    - 1/4 cup witch hazel astringent (you can use apple cider vinegar instead for acne-prone or oily skin to help adjust skin pH)
    - 1/4 cup lavender hydrosol
    - 2 tablespoons aloe vera juice or gel
    - For dry skin, add 2 teaspoons vegetable glycerin
    - 20 drops lavender essential oil. For problem skin, substitute tea tree oil.

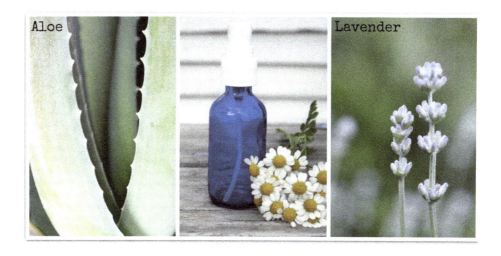

You Will Need:

- Measuring cup
- Glass jar with tight-fitting lid
- Blender
- Glass bottle for the finished toner. I like to use a spray bottle for easy application.
- Labels

Directions:

1. Mix all ingredients together and blend well.
2. Store in a glass jar.
3. Shake well before using.
4. Apply the toner after washing and gently drying your face.
5. There is no need to rinse this toner off before applying lotion or cream.
6. Lavender Face Toner can also be sprayed on any part of the body to add moisture before using a lotion bar, body butter, or balm.

Nourishing Lotion

Making your own lotion is easier than you think. This natural lotion is an emulsion, a rich blend of oils, waters and an emulsifier that are highly nourishing to the skin. An emulsion is a thorough blend of one liquid onto another, which are generally not compatible, such as oil and water. Lotion emulsions can grow mold, so remember to keep your working area really clean, sterilize all jars and equipment, and store your extra lotion in the refrigerator. You can add specialty fixed oils and essential oils to treat conditions such as dry skin, eczema, fungal infections, aging skin, etc. This recipe can be used on both the face and body.

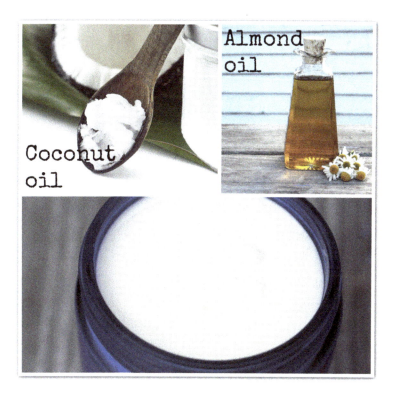

Ingredients:

Oil-based ingredients:

- Measure by volume:
    - 1 cup almond oil (or herbal oil such as calendula or comfrey)
    - 1/2 cup olive oil (or herbal oil)
    - 2 teaspoons lanolin
    - ½ teaspoon vitamin E oil or 1 ¼ teaspoon rosemary antioxidant
    - ½ teaspoon lavender essential oil
    - ½ teaspoon geranium essential oil
    - You can also add small amounts of specialty oils such as rosehip seed oil, jojoba, evening primrose, borage, avocado, walnut, neem, etc. These oils each have enriching, healing properties for the skin.
- Measure by weight:
    - 4 ounces coconut oil
    - 1 ounce beeswax

Water-based ingredients:

- Measure by volume:
    - 1 cup distilled water (or strong antioxidant tea)
    - 1/2 cup lavender hydrosol (or another of your preference)
    - 1/2 cup aloe vera gel
    - ½ teaspoon citric acid

You Will Need:

- Scale
- Large bowl
- Measuring cups and spoons
- Double boiler
- Blender

- Spatula
- Jars
- Labels

Directions:

1. Make sure all utensils and tools are disinfected before use.
2. Combine all "water" ingredients in a bowl and set aside.
3. You can add 1 teaspoon arrowroot powder to the water-based ingredients if you would like a lotion with a little less oily feel to it. Whisk well until fully incorporated.
4. In a double boiler, melt the beeswax.
5. Add the almond oil, olive oil, coconut oil, lanolin, and vitamin E oil to the double boiler and heat until melted. Stir well.
6. Pour the oils into a blender and let them cool to room temperature.
7. When the oil is at room temperature, add the essential oils.
8. After all ingredients have come to room temperature, you can begin mixing.
9. Turn the blender on high and slowly drizzle in the "water" ingredients until the water is no longer blending in well, or the mixture gets too thick to blend.
10. Sometimes more of the water mixture can be mixed into the emulsion by hand.
11. Pour into sterilized jars. I like to use a glass pump bottle so I don't put my hands in the lotion and increase the risk of contamination.
12. Let cool completely before capping.
13. Store extra in the refrigerator.
14. This rich recipe can be used on the face or the body.

Blemish Buster Balm

This treatment can be applied directly to any blemish, pimple, or infected area of the skin. I like using a roller ball applicator for the ease of application, although you should be careful not to spread an infection from one area of the skin to another.

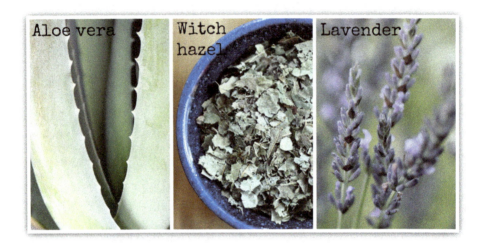

Ingredients:
- Measure by volume:
    - 1 tablespoon witch hazel astringent
    - 1 teaspoon aloe vera gel
    - 1/4 teaspoon vegetable glycerin (optional for drier skin)
    - 30 drops tea tree essential oil
    - 30 drops lavender essential oil
    - 10 drops *Eucalyptus radiata* essential oil

You Will Need:
- Spoon
- Bowl
- Label
- Glass dropper

- Glass bottle with roll on top

Directions:
1. Add all ingredients together in a bowl and mix well.
2. With your glass dropper, fill your roll-on bottle.
3. Apply as needed.
4. Store any extra in the refrigerator in a small glass bottle.

Beat the Heat Spray

This is an excellent mist for any time you feel hot. Whether it is a hot summer day, you have a fever, or during a hot flash, this blend is sure to cool you off!

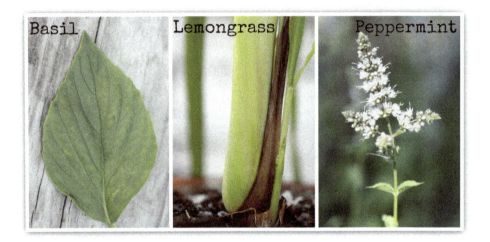

Ingredients:

- Measure by volume:
    - 4 ounces peppermint hydrosol
    - 16 drops peppermint essential oil
    - 16 drops basil essential oil
    - 8 drops lemongrass essential oil

You Will Need:

- Glass spray bottle
- Label

Directions:

1. Add all ingredients together in a glass bottle.
2. Shake well and spritz on your face and body any time you want a little cooling off.
3. Keep Beat the Heat Spray in the refrigerator, in your car, or take it with you during physical exertion. Be cool!

Gentle Exfoliating Grains

When exfoliating the skin of rough, dead skin, it is important to be very gentle. If we scrub too hard, we can expose immature skin cells that are not ready to do the important job of protecting our bodies from the environment around us. Instead, use a very light, circular touch, like a gentle massage. Gentle Exfoliating Grains can be used anywhere on the body to stimulate the skin and lymph, and for gentle exfoliation.

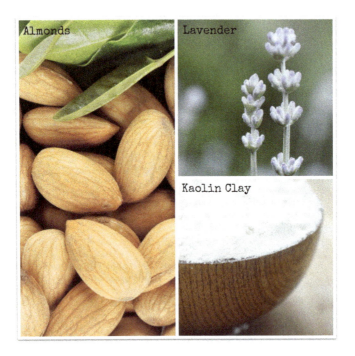

Ingredients:

- Measure by volume:
    - 2 cups kaolin clay
    - 1 cup rolled oats
    - 1/2 cup almonds
    - 1/8 cup lavender flowers
    - 1/8 cup calendula petals

- 40 drops lavender essential oil
- 20 drops geranium essential oil

You Will Need:

- Measuring cup
- Large bowl
- Blender or coffee grinder
- Containers
- Labels

Directions:

1. Combine oats, lavender, and calendula in a blender or coffee grinder and blend well.
2. Mix with kaolin clay.
3. Store in a well-sealed glass jar.
4. To use, take one tablespoon of Gentle Exfoliating Grains and moisten with a small amount of warm water, fixed oil, yogurt, or lavender or rose hydrosol.
5. Wet the face and massage in small gentle circles over the face, neck, or even the entire body!
6. Keep any extra in the refrigerator or freezer.

Fruity Facemask

This gentle, moisturizing recipe is excellent for helping to rebalance the skin after using harsh skin care products or face astringents high in alcohol. It is deeply nourishing and gently exfoliating to the skin.

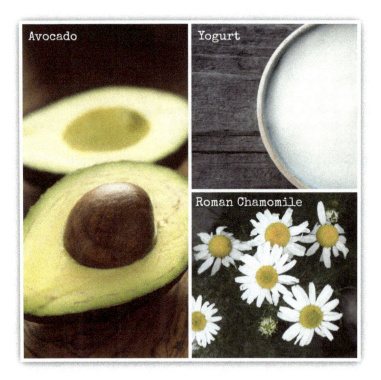

Ingredients:

- Measure by volume:
    - 2 tablespoons fresh fleshy fruit (such as papaya, apricot, peach, or pear)
    - 1 tablespoon fresh avocado
    - 3 teaspoons plain yogurt
    - 1 teaspoon jojoba oil (helpful for those with dry skin)
    - 1 teaspoon honey
    - 2 drops Roman chamomile essential oil

You Will Need:

- Measuring spoons
- Blender
- Bowl

Directions:

1. Mix all ingredients in a blender.
2. Transfer to a bowl before applying.
3. Apply mixture to face and neck and let sit for 15 to 20 minutes.
4. Then rinse– so refreshing!
5. If you have any leftover mask it can be stored in the refrigerator for a couple of days, shared with a friend, or composted.

Minty Tooth Powder

This tooth powder is very cleansing, restorative, and healing to the mouth, teeth, and gums. If you have only used toothpaste, this powder can take some getting used to, but once you do, you will love it!

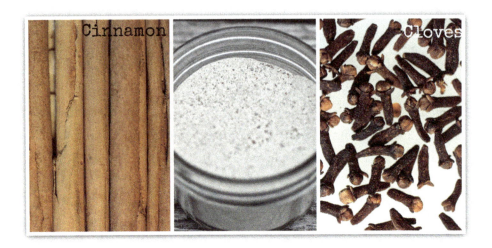

Ingredients:
- Measure by volume:
    - 4 tablespoons bentonite clay
    - 2 tablespoons calcium powder
    - 1 tablespoon magnesium powder
    - 1 tablespoon baking soda
    - 1 tablespoon sea salt, finely ground
    - 1 tablespoon cinnamon powder
    - 1 tablespoon myrrh gum powder
    - 1 teaspoon clove powder
    - 1 teaspoon powdered stevia herb, or 1 tablespoon xylitol (optional if you want a sweeter taste)
    - 50–70 drops peppermint or spearmint essential oil
    - 10 drops cinnamon essential oil

You Will Need:

- Blender or coffee grinder
- Bowl
- Glass jar or squeeze top bottle
- Label

Directions:

1. Powder any herbs such as whole cloves buds if necessary.
2. Mix all the ingredients in a bowl.
3. Store in a small jar with a lid or use a squeeze top bottle to apply the powder.
4. Wet your toothbrush before applying the powder and brush your teeth as you normally would.

My Favorite Lip Balm Recipe

I have to admit, I am a lip balm snob. I like just a certain consistency and feel, as well as liking my lip balms to last on my lips for a while. This is a wonderful and versatile recipe to make your own lip balm. You can play with it to create your own blend by adding different fixed vegetable oils, butters or essential oils. You can also add mica for a little shimmer, an herbal colorant such as alkanet or annatto, or even mineral oxides to make your own lipstick!

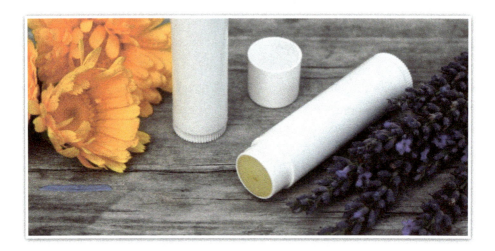

Ingredients:

- Measure by volume:
    - 3 ounces almond oil
    - 1 ounce jojoba oil
    - 1 ounce castor oil
    - ½ teaspoon vitamin E oil
    - ½ teaspoon essential oils such as rosemary, lavender, peppermint or spearmint

- Measure by weight:
    - 7 ounces coconut oil
    - 2 ounces cocoa butter

- o   3 ounces beeswax

You Will Need:

- Lip balm containers or tubes
- Double boiler
- Metal spoon
- Small funnel to pour the oil into the lip balm tubes if desired. I prefer just using a glass Pyrex measuring cup with a spout.
- Glass Pyrex measuring cup
- Rubber band to hold lip balm tubes upright in a group
- Plastic pipettes can also be useful for putting the oil into lip balm tubes. Glass droppers will not work as they cool the oil too quickly, causing clogging.

Directions:

1. Melt the beeswax in a double boiler.
2. Once the beeswax is melted, add the almond, castor, jojoba, and vitamin E oils.
3. Stir with a metal spoon until beeswax and oils are both totally melted.
4. Remove from heat immediately and stir in mica or mineral oxides (if desired) and essential oil.
5. Pour into your containers. Using a Pyrex measuring cup works best.
6. If using lip balm tubes, you can avoid creating a hole down the center of the tube by first filling the tubes 2/3 of the way up. Let them cool and then finish filling the tube. I like to hold my tubes upright by grouping them together with a rubber band.
7. This is a large recipe. Keep any extra lip balm in a glass jar in the refrigerator. When your lip balm is all used up, you can reuse your lip balm containers by melting the extra and pouring it into your old, well-cleaned lip balm containers.

Lovely Lips Balm

I created this simplified lip balm recipe for my niece as a do-it-yourself birthday present. This recipe makes a wonderful gift and is a fun "kit" to put together for anyone just getting interested in herbs or natural body care as well as any young person in your life. They are a huge hit at birthday parties!

Ingredients:

- Measure by volume:
    - 3 ounces almond oil
    - 1 ounce jojoba oil
    - 1 teaspoon castor oil
    - ½ teaspoon vitamin E oil
    - 1/4 ounce alkanet root or annatto (to give the lip balm a rose color if you wish)
    - 1/2 teaspoon sericite mica powder (to make your lip balm shiny if desired)
    - 40 drops of your favorite essential oil (don't use citrus oils as they are photosensitizing). I like peppermint, lavender, spearmint, or rosemary.
- Measure by weight:
    - 1 ounce beeswax

You Will Need:

- Coffee filter to filter the alkanet root out of the oil
- Lip balm containers or tubes
- Strainer
- Bowl
- Double boiler
- Metal spoon
- Small funnel to pour the oil into the lip balm tubes if desired

- Glass Pyrex measuring cup (or something to pour the lip balm with)
- Plastic pipettes can also be useful for putting the oil into lip balm tubes. Glass droppers will not work as they cool the oil too quickly, causing clogging.

Directions:

1. If you are using alkanet root, add it to the almond oil and let sit for 2 hours.
2. With alkanet root: Put the coffee filter in a strainer and set it over a bowl. Pour the oil through the coffee filter to strain out the alkanet root.
3. Add almond, jojoba, castor, and vitamin E oils together and mix well.
4. Melt the beeswax in a double boiler.
5. Once the beeswax is melted, add the fixed oils.
6. Stir with a metal spoon until beeswax and oils are both totally melted.
7. Remove from heat immediately and stir in mica or mineral oxides (if desired) and essential oil.
8. Pour into your containers. Using a Pyrex measuring cup works best.
9. If using lip balm tubes, you can avoid creating a hole down the center of the tube by first filling the tubes 2/3 of the way up. Let them cool and then finish filling the tube. I like to hold my tubes upright by grouping them together with a rubber band.
10. Keep any extra lip balm in a glass jar in the refrigerator. When your lip balm is all used up, you can reuse your lip balm containers by melting the extra and pouring it into your old, well-cleaned lip balm containers.

Recipes for the Bath

Natural baths are a wonderful way to heal your body and rejuvenate your soul. Healing baths can be useful to encourage relaxation, detoxify the skin, relieve sore muscles, and ease achy joints. Baths can even help ease illnesses such as cold and flu by bringing blood to the surface of the skin and encouraging elimination through sweating. Most importantly, they are a way to take time for ourselves, reminding us to create a space to relax, pamper ourselves, prioritize our own wellbeing, and create an opportunity to recharge. Here are some recipes to help you make herbal bathing a tool for your own self-care! May they inspire you to take some time out, relax, and explore your senses. Breathe deeply, slow down, and feel your center.

> *I am sure there are things that can't be cured by a good bath but I can't think of one.*
> ~ Sylvia Plath

Before we start, a few quick suggestions about taking a bath. First, remember to hydrate! We may not notice, but taking a hot bath makes us sweat. For this reason, it is important to drink lots of water or herbal tea while in the tub. Second, although glass is by far the best receptacle when using essential oils in a bath blend, please be cautious using glass around the bath or shower, especially with children. Finally, be cautious when exiting the tub. Hot baths can make you lightheaded, and standing quickly can cause dizziness.

Blissful Bath

A blend of salt, herbs, and essential oils, this sublime bath is soothing to the skin and calming to the nerves. Stored in a clear glass jar, it is a delight just to look at this blend!

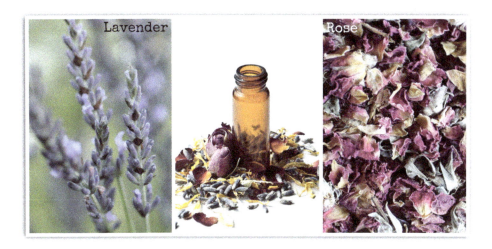

Ingredients:

- Measure by volume:
    - 1 cup chamomile flowers
    - 1 cup lavender flowers
    - 1 cup organic rolled oats
    - 1/2 cup rose flowers
    - 3 cups sea salt
    - 90 drops lavender essential oil
    - 30 drops marjoram essential oil
    - 20 drops clary sage essential oil
    - 10 drops ylang-ylang essential oil

You will need:

- Measuring cup
- Glass or stainless steel bowl
- Spoon
- Glass jars
- Labels
- Small muslin bag or large tea ball

Directions:

1. Mix all ingredients together in a large bowl.
2. Store in a glass jar.
3. To use, scoop 3 tablespoons of Blissful Bath into a muslin bag or large tea ball and add to the bath.
4. Sit back, read a good book or listen to some soothing music, and relax!

Stress Relief Bath

Feeling on edge and overwhelmed? Try this healing bath blend to calm and soothe. Stress Relief Bath blend makes a lovely evening bath, helpful for relaxing and useful for encouraging a restful sleep for both children and adults.

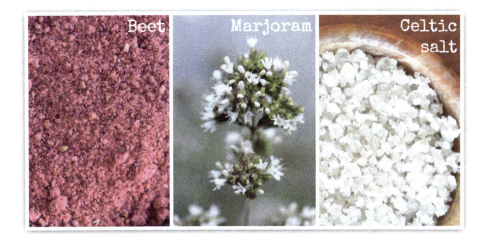

Ingredients:

- Measure by volume:
    - 2 cups Celtic sea salt
    - 1 tablespoon beet powder
    - 50 drops lavender essential oil
    - 25 drops clary sage essential oil
    - 25 drops marjoram essential oil

You Will Need:

- Measuring cup
- Measuring spoons
- Glass or stainless steel bowl
- Spoon

- Glass jar with tight-fitting lid
- Label

Directions:

1. Mix ingredients well and store in an airtight glass jar.
2. Unplug the phone and light a candle.
3. Put on some relaxing music.
4. Draw a hot bath and slip into it.
5. Add 2 tablespoons (1 tablespoon for a child) Stress Relief Bath Blend, sit back, and relax!

Rose Cream Bath

This decadent bath is hydrating and gently exfoliating the skin due to its high milk fat and lactic acid content. The aroma of rose adds a loving allure. For a romantic evening, it can make a sensual bath for two.

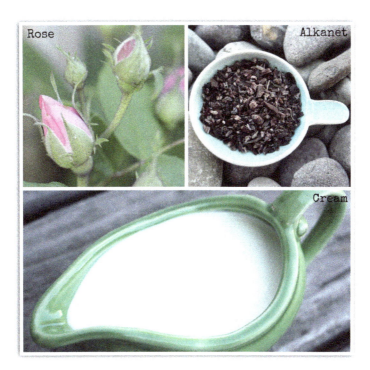

Ingredients:

- Measure by volume:
    - 1 cup fresh cream (or coconut milk)
    - 1 tablespoon alkanet root
    - 1 cup rose hydrosol or water
    - 5 drops rose essential oil
    - 10 drops geranium essential oil

You Will Need:

- Measuring cup
- Measuring spoons
- Glass or stainless steel bowl
- Spoon
- Strainer

Directions:

1. Add alkanet root to the cream.
2. Mix well.
3. Let sit for 2 hours to overnight and then strain.
4. Add the essential oils and rose water to the now pink cream and stir well.
5. Submerge yourself in a hot bath and add your Rose Cream Bath blend.
6. Massage this luxurious blend into your skin as you bathe.

Forest Grove Bath Melts

These bars are a simple blend of sweet almond oil, cocoa butter, and essential oil. You can add herbs or natural colors as well, or make them unscented by leaving out the essential oils (the cocoa butter itself smells like chocolate). Once in the bath, you can rub them on your skin for extra hydration. They leave your skin soft and silky and add a moisturizing element to the bath for dry, irritated skin or eczema.

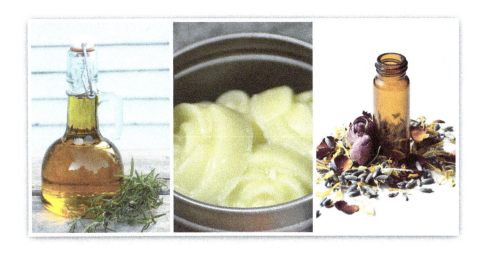

Ingredients:

- Measure by weight:
    - 8 ounces cocoa butter
- Measure by volume:
    - ½ cup sweet almond oil
    - 60 drops orange essential oil
    - 30 drops cedar essential oil
    - 30 drops fir essential oil

You Will Need:

- Scale
- Measuring cup
- Double boiler
- Spoon
- Molds
- Glass jars or containers
- Labels

Directions:

1. In a double boiler, melt the cocoa butter.
2. Add the almond oil and stir until melted.
3. Remove from the burner and add the essential oils. At this point, you can also add some dried lavender flowers, rose petals, calendula blossoms, or natural colorant if you wish.
4. Pour into molds and let cool completely. I find that small glycerin soap molds work well, but you can also use small muffin pans or candy molds. This recipe takes a while to cool and solidify. You can put the molds in the refrigerator to speed the process.
5. To use, get in the tub, add a bath melt and watch it melt. Kids love this part!
6. Gently rub the oils into your skin.
7. Be careful when exiting the tub as the oil can make surfaces slippery!

Sleepy Baby Bath

Herbal baths are one of my favorite ways to use medicinal plants with infants. With babies six months or younger it is always important to use gentle herbs and stay away from most essential oils. This blend is helpful to encourage restful sleep for any small child before naptime or bed. It will also help soothe colic or an upset tummy.

Ingredients:

- Measure by volume:
    - ½ cup chamomile flowers
    - ½ cup lavender flowers
    - ½ cup catnip herb

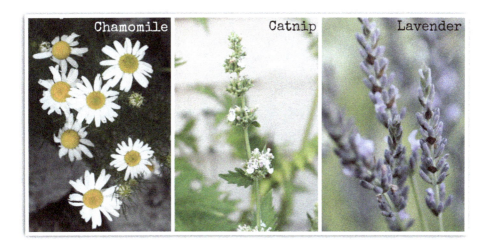

You Will Need:

- Measuring cup
- Bowl
- Teakettle or pan
- Tablespoon
- Teapot or quart canning jar

- Strainer
- Glass jar
- Label

Directions:

1. Mix herbs in a bowl and store in a glass jar.
2. Pour 2 cups of boiling water over 2 tablespoons of the herbal blend and let steep until cool.
3. Strain and add the tea to baby's bath water.
4. There is no need to rinse this blend off.

Detox Vinegar Bath

This bath is excellent to use if you are fasting, doing a cleanse, or have a cold or flu, or to prepare your body for the change of each season.

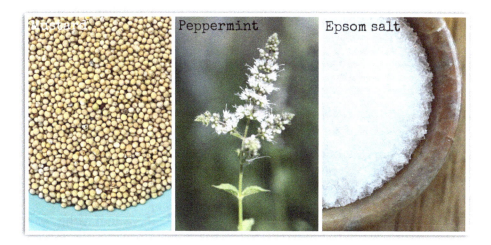

Ingredients:

- Measure by volume:
    - 1 tablespoon freshly ground mustard seed
    - 1 tablespoon freshly ground sage leaf
    - ½ cup Epsom salt
    - ¼ cup bentonite clay
    - 30 drops eucalyptus essential oil
    - 30 drops rosemary essential oil
    - 30 drops peppermint essential oil
    - ½ cup apple cider vinegar

You Will Need:

- Blender, coffee grinder or a mortar and pestle
- Glass or stainless steel bowl
- Measuring cup
- Measuring spoons

Directions:

1. Grind your mustard seed and sage leaf in a blender, coffee grinder or with a mortar and pestle.
2. In a bowl, mix the Epsom salt, clay, mustard seed, and sage leaf powder together.
3. Add the essential oils and mix well.
4. Get in a hot bath, and add all ingredients to the bath, including the vinegar.
5. Soak for at least 20 minutes.
6. To aid in the cleansing process, be sure to drink plenty of water or herbal tea during and after your bath.

Herbal Bath Bombs

These skin-softening bombs make a lovely, fizzy, scent-filled addition to any bath! They are particularly fun for children (and the young at heart). Bath bombs make great gifts!

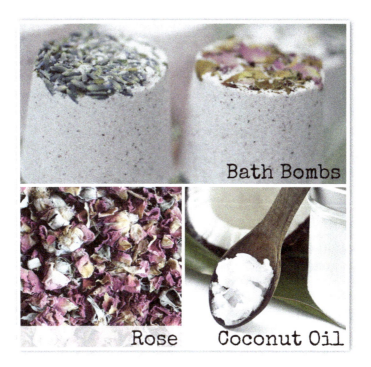

Ingredients:

- Measure by volume:
    - 1 cup citric acid
    - 2 cups baking soda
    - 2 tablespoons coconut oil
    - Natural colorant of your choice (start with 1 teaspoon)
    - 2–3 teaspoons (10–15 mLs) essential oil(s) of your choice
    - Witch hazel or rose hydrosol
    - Herbs such as lavender, rose, rosemary, and calendula

You Will Need:

- Measuring cup
- Measuring spoons
- Blender
- Large glass or stainless steel bowl
- Large fork or dough cutter
- Squirt bottle
- Spoon
- Molds (candy molds, glycerin soap molds, small paper cups, or mini muffin tins work well)

Directions:

1. Blend the citric acid and baking soda together thoroughly. This step is very important—if you don't blend well, you end up with a grainy bomb. Use a mixer with larger batches.
2. With a large fork or dough cutter, work the coconut oil into the citric acid and baking soda until the mixture looks like cornmeal. Having some larger chunks of coconut oil is OK.
3. Once you've blended the above ingredients really well, add your colorant and herbs if desired. Don't add too much though—the color shows up once you add the witch hazel.
4. Add essential oils to your personal preference. You will need 2–3 teaspoons depending on how much aroma you want.
5. Now, this is the difficult part. Spritz (with a squirt bottle) the witch hazel or hydrosol onto your batch while stirring with the other hand. Kids love to help with this! Watch for bubbling, a sign that you are adding too much liquid to a certain area.
6. When your batch sticks together when squeezed, you need to start putting it in molds.

7. Time is of the essence; if you wait too long, the mixture will get hard. If you spritz too much, the mixture will be too wet and start the fizzing reaction.
8. Put the bombs in molds. You can add some herbs into the bottom of the mold first if you wish.
9. The harder you pack the bath bombs, the denser, heavier, and more durable they will be.
10. Wait a few minutes and tap them out.
11. Let them air dry for 3 or 4 hours and voilà: wonderful, hard bath bombs.
12. To use one, get into a warm bath and add the bath bomb. Watch it fizz and enjoy the healing benefits.

Sore Foot Soak

This soak invigorates sore, tired feet. It is valuable for ingrown toenails, bacterial infections, and fungal infections such as athlete's foot or toenail fungus. You can sprinkle this blend into shoes to reduce odor. To avoid a mess, make sure to shake your shoes out before wearing.

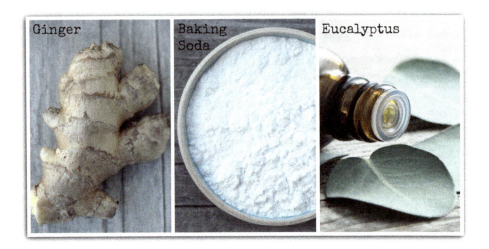

Ingredients:

- Measure by volume:
    - 1 cup baking soda
    - 1 cup Epsom salt
    - 1 tablespoon powdered ginger root
    - 30 drops tea tree essential oil
    - 30 drops peppermint essential oil
    - 30 drops *Eucalyptus globulus* essential oil

You Will Need:

- Measuring cup
- Measuring spoons

- Glass or stainless steel bowl
- Spoon
- Glass jars
- Labels

Directions:

1. In a bowl, mix all ingredients together.
2. Store in a glass jar with a tight-fitting lid.
3. In a tub of hot water (not too hot!), add 2 tablespoons of Sore Foot Soak.
4. Mix well.
5. Immerse feet, sit back, and relax with a cup of herbal tea.
6. Soak feet for at least 10 minutes.
7. To use for deodorizing and refreshing shoes, simply sprinkle 1–2 tablespoons in each shoe and shake well. Let sit for 2 hours and empty out. Waterproof sandals can be soaked in 4 cups of water infused with 4 tablespoons Sore Foot Soak.

Sinus Steam

Oddly enough, the sore foot soak can also be a useful addition to a sinus steam. To do this, get a pot of steaming water (not boiling) and remove it from the stove. Set it on a safe surface. Place your face over the water. Drape a towel over your head and around the pot to hold in the steam. Place a teaspoon of the salts into the water, close your eyes, and breathe deeply through your nose. You can repeat this process several times to reduce nasal congestion and sooth sinus infection.

For a small child, drape a blanket over an umbrella and sit underneath with them. Carefully slide in your hot water and add your Sore Foot Soak. Be careful that the child does not touch the pan or hot water.

Ache No More Bath

This bath blend can be helpful to reduce soreness and recovery time after exercise, physical accident or injury, or to aid the stiffness from arthritis or achy joints.

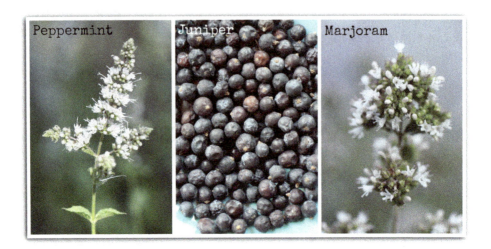

Ingredients:
- Measure by volume:
    - 1 cup Epsom salt
    - 1 cup baking soda
    - ½ cup willow bark
    - 20 drops birch essential oil (don't use with blood thinning medications)
    - 20 drops marjoram essential oil
    - 20 drops rosemary essential oil
    - 20 drops juniper essential oil
    - 10 drops peppermint essential oil

You Will Need:

- Measuring cup
- Glass or stainless steel bowl
- Spoon
- Glass jars
- Labels

Directions:

1. Mix all ingredients well in a bowl.
2. Store in a glass jar with a tight-fitting lid.
3. Add ¼ cup salts to an old sock or muslin bag.
4. Fill the bath with warm water, get in and add your salts.
5. Soak for at least 20 minutes.
6. Rinse off after your bath and rub vigorously, rubbing toward your heart as you dry. This movement helps circulate the lymph and remove waste products from sore muscles and joints.

Scentual Bath

This alluring bath blend is a relaxing bath for one or a romantic bath for two. Placed in a beautiful jar, this blend makes a wonderful wedding gift, Valentine's Day present, or a fun recipe to spice up your love life.

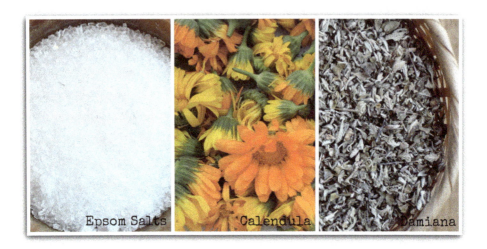

Ingredients:

- Measure by volume:
    - 1 cup Epsom salt
    - 1 cup sea salt
    - 1 cup baking soda
    - ½ cup rolled oats
    - ½ cup lavender buds
    - ½ cup calendula flowers
    - ½ cup rose petals
    - ½ cup damiana herb
    - 60 drops rosewood essential oil
    - 30 drops ylang-ylang essential oil
    - 10 drops blood orange essential oil

You Will Need:

- Glass or stainless steel bowl
- Measuring cup
- Spoon
- Glass jars
- Labels

Directions:

1. Mix ingredients well and store in an airtight glass jar.
2. Add 2 tablespoons per bath into a muslin bag, large tea ball, old sock, or cloth tied with string.

Wake Me Up Bath

This stimulating blend invigorates and encourages alertness. Wake Me Up Bath can be used in the morning as a bath salt, or you can add a fixed oil to it and use it as a body scrub.

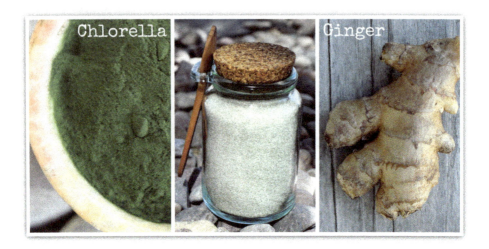

Ingredients:

- Measure by volume:
    - 1 cup finely ground Celtic sea salt
    - ¼ cup ginger powder
    - 1 teaspoon chlorella powder
    - 25 drops fir essential oil
    - 25 drops grapefruit essential oil
    - 25 drops orange essential oil

You Will Need:

- Measuring cup
- Measuring spoons
- Glass or stainless steel bowl

- Spoon
- Glass jars
- Labels

Directions:

1. Add the Celtic sea salt, ginger powder, and chlorella powder together in a bowl and mix well.
2. Add all essential oils and combine thoroughly.
3. Store in a glass jar with a tight-fitting lid.
4. After submerging yourself in a hot bath, add two tablespoons Wake Me Up Bath to the tub for a refreshing pick me up.

WAKE ME UP SCRUB

1. If you want to make a body scrub, add a fixed oil to your jar of salts until there is ¼ inch of oil covering the salts.
2. Add 1 teaspoon vitamin E oil to help preserve your scrub.
3. After using the body scrub, rinse well, and gently pat dry.

Recipes for the Hair

Our hair helps to protect our head and keep it warm. Hair is the fastest normally growing tissue in the body. It grows an average of one-half inch per month. The main component of human hair is a protein called keratin, which is also found in the skin, teeth, fingernails, and toenails. Although it is normal to lose hair, increased hair loss can occur due to hormonal changes, increased stress levels, dieting, or severe shock.

Our hair is alive and growing inside the hair follicle. Blood vessels in the follicle nourish the hair and encourage proper hair growth. Although the hair that we see on the top of our head is considered dead, it can reflect our general health and wellbeing. Having healthy hair, skin, and nails is a good indicator of overall health. People with nutritional deficiencies tend to have dry, dull hair, and sometimes experience high levels of hair loss. Nutrients that encourage healthy hair growth include protein, iron, zinc, vitamin D, omega-3 fatty acids, B vitamins, biotin, and vitamin C.

Harsh hair products, dyes, blow dryers, and curling irons can damage the hair. Similar to our skin, our scalp needs a balance of oils and microorganisms to be healthy. It is important to use gentle products on the hair so as to not to strip the scalp or hair shaft and keep the hair and scalp nourished and moisturized.

> *True beauty comes from inside. It comes from our actions and our interactions.*

Horsetail Hair Rinse

This rinse is wonderful to maintain healthy hair and scalp. Use Horsetail Hair Rinse once a week to encourage a proper pH balance, remove mineral and chemical buildup in the hair, and add shine.

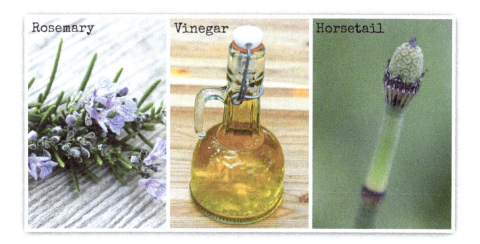

Ingredients:

- Measure by volume:
    - 2 cups apple cider
    - 1 cup water or hydrosol (I recommend chamomile or rosemary hydrosol)
    - ¼ cup horsetail herb
    - ¼ cup nettles leaves
    - ¼ cup rosemary leaves
    - ¼ cup chamomile flowers
    - 1 teaspoon essential oil of your choice. I recommend peppermint to stimulate circulation, rosemary for dark hair, chamomile for blond hair, or tea tree for scalp itchiness or dandruff.

You Will Need:

- Measuring cup
- Measuring spoons
- Glass jar with a tight-fitting lid
- Strainer
- Glass spray bottle (always be careful with glass in the shower)
- Label

Directions:

1. Add herbs to a glass jar and pour apple cider vinegar and water or hydrosol over the top.
2. Let sit for 2 weeks to one month and strain.
3. Add your essential oils.
4. Pour in a glass spray bottle.
5. After washing the hair, shake Vinegar Herbal Hair Rinse well and spray on the hair and scalp.
6. Let sit 2–5 minutes, rinse and shine!

Natural Lice Treatments

Many people are reluctant to use insecticidal head lice treatments on themselves and their family. Natural remedies can work just as well, or sometimes even better. Most over-the-counter treatments contain malathion or pyrethroid, products which seem to be becoming less effective, possibly because head lice have become resistant to these insecticides. When treating head lice naturally, there are some generally recommended practices that will reduce the risk of reinfestation.

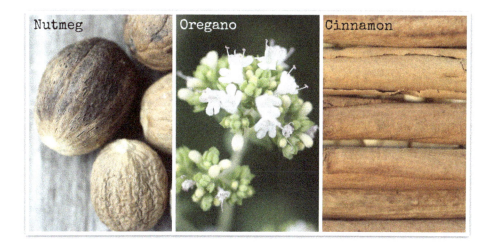

In General:

1. Vacuum thoroughly, and daily.
2. Wash clothes, sheets, hats, coats, etc. in hot water and dry them completely on high heat.
3. If you can't wash an article of clothing, or item, seal it in a plastic bag for 10 days. This will kill the lice, as they have no access to food.
4. Comb your hair with a lice comb to get out dying lice and eggs, also called nits.
5. Adding heat also helps to kill the lice. You can accomplish this by using a blow dryer after applying your herbal formula to increase the effectiveness of the natural lice treatments.

Below is a list of natural treatments and essential oils that have been researched for their effectiveness in killing both adult lice as well as their nits. I created this recipe when my boys brought head lice home from school and it worked very well! I have since shared it with many people who have had similar results.

Ingredients:

- Cinnamon leaf essential oil
- Tea tree essential oil
- Peppermint essential oil
- Nutmeg essential oil
- Oregano essential oil
- Anise essential oil
- Red thyme essential oil
- Optional ingredients:
    - Vodka
    - Apple cider vinegar
    - Water
    - Olive oil (or another fixed oil)

You Will Need:

- Measuring cup
- Glass dropper
- Glass bottles, include a spray bottle if you make the Lice Spray recipe
- Label

Directions:

You can combine any of the below recipes for your natural lice treatment. I prefer using all of them together.

Lice Spray

1. Take 1 ounce (30mL) vodka and mix it with 7 drops (one of each oil) of the above essential oils.
2. Spray liberally onto the scalp. Be careful to avoid the eyes and other sensitive areas. Rub in and leave on overnight.
3. Wash the spray off in the morning with shampoo.
4. Finish with the Lice Rinse.
5. Repeat the treatment after 1 week.
6. This spray can also be used on bedding, pillows, furniture, clothing, backpacks, etc. to deter lice.

Lice Rinse

1. Make a mixture of 1 tablespoon apple cider vinegar and 1 tablespoon water.
2. Mix with 7 drops (one of each) of essential oil.
3. Use this as a rinse liberally after washing hair.
4. Do not rinse out.
5. Repeat the treatment after 1 week.

Lice Oil

1. Take 1 ounce (30ml) olive oil and mix it with 7 drops (one of each) of the above essential oils.
2. Rub liberally into the scalp and leave on overnight.
3. Make sure to cover your pillow with an old towel.
4. Wash the oil off in the morning with shampoo.
5. Finish with the Lice Rinse.
6. Repeat the treatment after 1 week.

Healthy Hair Oil

This blend of fixed and essential oils preserves moisture and replenishes the hair. It encourages circulation to the scalp, which in turn brings nutrients to the hair follicle. You can customize the essential oils for this formula based on your hair color and scalp health.

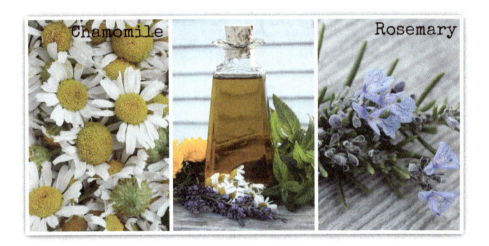

Ingredients:

- Measure by volume:
    - ¼ cup almond oil
    - ¼ cup jojoba oil
    - 1 tablespoon avocado oil
    - ¼ teaspoon vitamin E Oil

You Will Need:

- Glass jar or pump bottle
- Label
- Measuring cup
- Measuring spoons

Directions:

1. Mix all ingredients together in a jar and shake well.
2. Store in a dark glass pump bottle for easy application.
3. To apply, pump a small amount into your hand.
4. With your fingertips, massage the oil into the scalp.
5. Let the oil sit for 20 minutes or even leave on overnight.
6. If left on overnight, be sure to cover your pillow with an old towel.
7. To remove, use a natural shampoo, first applied to the hair without water.
8. Add water and wash well.
9. You may need two washings to remove the oil.

Healthy Hair Oil Variations:

You can add different ingredients to the above recipe for specific hair or scalp conditions listed below.

Dandruff or Fungal Infection of the Scalp

- ¼ teaspoon neem oil
- 40 drops tea tree essential oil

Hair Growth

- 20 drops rosemary essential oil
- 20 drops cedar essential oil

Dark Hair

- 40 drops rosemary essential oil

Light Hair

- 40 drops Roman chamomile essential oil

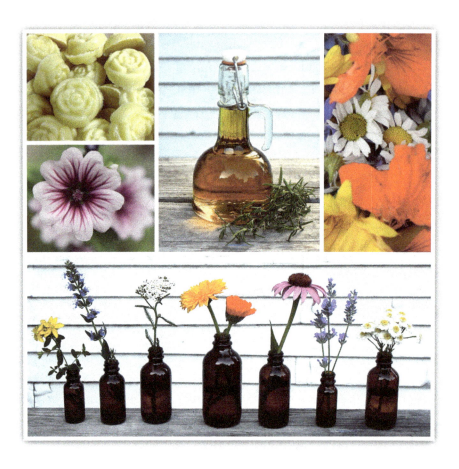

No More Flakes

Tired of those embarrassing flakes? They are actually trying to tell you that your scalp is out of balance. Seborrheic dermatitis is an inflammatory, itchy skin condition that causes flaky, white to yellowish scales to form on oily areas such as the scalp or inside the ear. Here are some great natural tips to end the flakes! A dandruff home remedy needs to be used for a prolonged period of time to ensure that the condition is successfully treated. Use these suggestions for a minimum of 2 weeks to see lasting results.

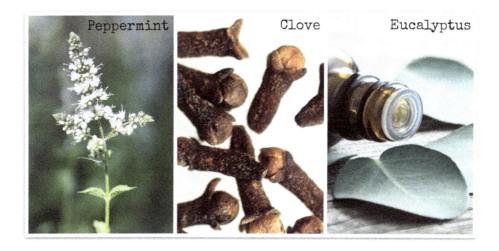

In general:

1. Don't use harsh shampoos or chemical styling products such as gels or hairspray.
2. Do not expose the scalp to extreme temperatures such as blow dryers, showers that are too hot, or curling irons close to the scalp.
3. Make sure you are having a daily bowel movement. Bowel health has a direct effect on skin health.
4. Take two tablespoons of fenugreek seeds and soak them overnight in water. Strain and grind them into a fine paste in the morning. This paste should be applied all over the scalp and left for half an hour. Use this

treatment twice a week for the first two weeks and then once a week for another two weeks.
5. Use a teaspoon of fresh lime juice for the last rinse after washing the hair. This not only leaves the hair glowing but also removes stickiness and prevents dandruff. Lime juice or lemon juice is an excellent oily dandruff home remedy. Let the juice sit for 2 minutes and then rinse well.
6. Brush hair daily. This helps to stimulate circulation and keep the scalp healthy.
7. Choose natural shampoos and conditioners. Avoid sulfates, parabens, synthetic fragrances, and petrochemicals.
8. Take an essential fatty acid supplement to increase the oil balance on the skin.

Ingredients:

- Measure by volume:
    - 2 ounces ethyl alcohol (or Everclear). Jojoba oil can be used as a substitute if you have dry hair or scalp.
    - 14 drops peppermint essential oil
    - 12 drops camphor essential oil
    - 12 drops clove essential oil
    - 12 drops *Eucalyptus globulus* essential oil

You Will Need:

- Measuring cup
- Glass dropper
- Glass bottle or jar with a tight-fitting lid
- Label

Directions:

1. Mix all ingredients together and store in a glass bottle or jar.
2. Before washing the hair, apply this treatment to the scalp and let it sit for 20 minutes. Be careful to avoid the eyes and other sensitive areas.
3. Apply shampoo to the hair before wetting.
4. Wash hair as you normally would. If using jojoba oil, you may need to shampoo twice.
5. Do this 3 times a week for a minimum of 2 weeks, then twice a week for the next 2 weeks.
6. Say hello to a healthier scalp!

In Closing

The body is sacred. Part of being healthy is learning to love ourselves, in all of our imperfection. When we think of our bodies, we often think of what we wish were different. We wish we were thinner, or less wrinkled, that our nose was smaller or our lips were bigger. We wish we were taller or shorter or more... something or less... something else.

What if you are actually just perfect and beautiful the way you are? What if you really believed that? How would your life be different? Although this isn't necessarily easy to believe, I think it a worthy idea to practice. By that, I mean to make the effort to think differently about your own body, praise it, tell it all the good things about it, love it and appreciate it for everything it does for you. Our bodies enable us to experience and move through the world. They are a way we feel pleasure, breathe, and assimilate nutrients, and eliminate wastes. Our bodies allow most of us to smell, taste, hear, see, and interact with our surroundings.

> *Dare to love yourself as if you were a rainbow with gold at both ends.*
> ~ Aberjhani

Let us remember to love and appreciate our amazing bodies. Ultimately, self-love nourishes our body *and* our spirit. Most importantly, no matter what, may we be gentle and kind to ourselves, eliminating that inner voice of self-criticism. May we acknowledge our efforts, love ourselves for all the good we see and do and are. May we accept our flaws and the fact that we are all are beautifully imperfect. May we all remember that true beauty comes from inside. It comes from our actions and our interactions.

A Blessing for the Body
Cleansing Ritual, Breath of Healing

by Karrie Westwood

The bath or shower is a wonderful gift to give yourself. It is one of the few times in a busy day you can be completely alone with your thoughts and your breath. It is a perfect time to connect with your divine self and honor your self for all you are and do each day. So next time you are getting prepared to step into your bath, shower, or even your daily facial cleansing regime, give yourself three breaths. First start by completely releasing any air you are holding onto. Completely exhale from the deepest darkest cells of your lungs as you step into the bath or shower, or as you look into the mirror.

As you take your first deep breath, breathe in the love of the Divine Mother: the love that is all around you waiting to nurture you and soothe your tired soul.

Exhale all that you are holding, any anger, pain, or discomfort in your body. Let it all go!

As you take your next breath, breathe in deeply and feel the water as it flows over your body and surrounds you in Universal Compassion, compassion for your deepest darkest places.

Exhale any fears or concerns all the way down to your toes.

As you take your next deep breath fill your lungs with all the joy they can hold. Life is a lesson and we choose how to learn it in Joy or Sorrow. Choose Joy!

May each breath be filled with love, compassion, and joy for yourself and all those you come in contact with.

Index

A

abrasions · 79
  aloe vera · 22
acacia gum · 52
Acacia sp. · 52
acne · 114, 116
  aloe vera · 22
  apple cider vinegar · 55
  cedar essential oil · 38
  chlorophyll · 34
  cranberry · 34
  eucalyptus essential oil · 38
  Fuller's earth · 30
  geranium essential oil · 38
  hazelnut oil · 45
  neem · 45
  oats · 57
  orange essential oil · 39
  rosehip seed oil · 46
  sea buckthorn oil · 46
  tea tree essential oil · 40
  turmeric · 34
  yogurt · 59
advertising · 72
agrimony · 20, 68
alkanet root · 32, 7091, 134, 135, 141, 142
Alkanna tinctoria · 32
Allantoin · 23
allergic reactions · 18
almond oil · 44, 65, 70, 87, 88, 90, 91, 102, 103, 104, 105, 112, 113, 120, 121, 132, 134, 143, 144, 166
almonds · 102, 103, 126
Aloe barbadensis miller · 21
aloe vera · 20, 21, 65, 68, 70, 71, 77, 78, 117, 120, 122
anise essential oil · 164
annatto · 32, 68
antibacterial
  aloe vera · 22
  annatto · 32
  calendula · 22
  cinnamon essential oil · 38
  coconut oil · 49
  essential oils · 61
  geranium essential oil · 38
  neem · 45
  rose · 26
  tea tree essential oil · 40
  turmeric · 35
antifungal · 83
  apple cider vinegar · 55
  beet · 33
  calendula · 22
  cinnamon essential oil · 38
  coconut oil · 49
  geranium essential oil · 38
  neem · 45
  tea tree essential oil · 40
anti-inflammatory · 66
  aloe vera · 22
  beet · 33
  birch essential oil · 37
  chamomile · 23
  chlorophyll · 33
  eucalyptus essential oil · 38
  ginger · 24
  oats · 57
  rose · 26
  rose essential oil · 39
  rosemary antioxidant · 62
  self-heal · 27
  shea butter · 51
  turmeric · 34
  walnut oil · 47
anti-inflammatory herbs · 20
antimicrobial · 66, 83
  chlorophyll · 33
  cinnamon essential oil · 38
  coconut oil · 49
  essential oils · 36, 61
  honey · 56
  neem · 45
  peppermint essential oil · 39
  rosemary · 27
  rosemary antioxidant · 62
  sage · 27
antimicrobial herbs · 20
antioxidant · 19, 56, 60, 114, 120
  aloe vera · 22
  annatto · 33
  beet · 33
  cacao · 33
  chlorophyll · 33
  cinnamon essential oil · 38
  cocoa butter · 49
  coconut oil · 49
  cranberry · 34
  grape seed oil · 45

antioxidant *(cont.)*
   kokum butter · 50
   oats · 57
   olive oil · 46
   rose · 26
   rose essential oil · 39
   rosehip seed oil · 46
   rosemary · 27
   rosemary antioxidant · 62
   rosemary essential oil · 40
   sea buckthorn oil · 46
   sesame oil · 46
   shea butter · 51
   vitamin C · 58
   vitamin E · 62
   walnut oil · 47
antioxidant herbs · 60
antiseptic
   baking soda · 56
   orange essential oil · 39
   rose essential oil · 40
   rosemary essential oil · 40
   sea salt · 42
   self-heal · 27
antiviral
   cinnamon essential oil · 38
   lemon balm · 25
   tea tree essential oil · 40
apple cider vinegar · 55, 68, 117, 147, 148, 161, 162, 164, 165
apricot · 128
argan oil · 70
arnica · 20, 73, 81
arrowroot powder · 52, 70, 89, 107, 121
arthritis · 81, 154
   birch essential oil · 37
   Dead Sea salts · 42
artificial colorants · 18
ascorbic acid · 115, 116, *See* vitamin C
ascorbyl palmitate · *See* vitamin C
aspen · 20
Aspergillus niger · 61
astringent · 117, 122
   alkanet · 32
   annatto · 32
   cranberry · 34
   Epsom salt · 42
   grape seed oil · 45
   hazelnut oil · 45
   plantain · 26
   rose · 26
   rose essential oil · 40
   sage · 27
   self-heal · 27
Astringent herbs · 20
Avena sativa · 57
avocado · 56, 128
avocado oil · 44, 68, 70, 71, 95, 96, 112, 120, 166
Azadirachta indica · 45

B

baking soda · 56, 89, 130, 149, 150, 152, 154, 156
banana · 56
basil essential oil · 124
bay laurel essential oil · 93
bayberry · 20, 68
beeswax · 10, 52, 56, 79, 80, 81, 82, 84, 86, 87, 88, 120, 121, 133, 135
beet · 33, 65, 68, 70, 71, 139
bentonite clay · 29, 65, 68, 70, 71, 130, 147
Benzoin essential oil · 70, 93, 105
benzoin gum · 75, 76
Bergamot essential oil · 68, 105
Beta vulgaris · 33, 57
Betula spp. · 37
bilberry · 61, 70
birch essential oil · 37, 81, 154
Bixa orellana · 32
blackberry · 20
blemishes · 30
   chlorophyll · 34
   tea tree essential oil · 40
blond hair · 161
   chamomile · 23
blood orange essential oil · 156
blueberry · 56, 61, 71
body powder · 107
   arrowroot · 52
   bentonite clay · 29
   clays · 29
   cornstarch · 53
   Fuller's earth · 30
   tapioca starch · 58
body scrub · 41, 42, 105, 158, 159
borage oil · 71, 95, 96, 112, 120
borax · 56
Brassica spp. · 25
brazil nut oil · 70
brown sugar · 58, 105

bruises · 81
    comfrey · 23
    Epsom salt · 42
    marjoram essential oil · 39
bug bites · 89
    calendula · 22
    lavender · 24
    lavender essential oil · 38
    marjoram essential oil · 39
    plantain · 26
burns
    aloe vera · 22
    comfrey · 23
    geranium essential oil · 38
    lavender · 24
    lavender essential oil · 38
    marjoram essential oil · 39
    plantain · 25
    turmeric · 34

C

cacao · 33, 49, 61, 65, 68, 70, 71
calcium · 29, 30, 31, 42, 43, 130
    kelp · 24
calendula · 21, 22, 65, 68, 70, 71, 73, 79, 83, 98, 126, 149, 156
Calendula officinalis · 22
calming · 39, 137
    cedar essential oil · 38
    lavender · 24
    orange essential oil · 39
camphor essential oil · 81, 169
cardamom essential oil · 93, 105, 106
carnauba wax · 49, 53, 65, 70
carrier oils · 44, *See* fixed oils
carrot seed essential oil · 70, 71
carrot seed hydrosol · 71
castor oil · 93, 94, 132, 134
catnip · 145
cayenne · 21, 73
Cedar essential oil · 38, 68, 89, 143, 167
Cedrus spp. · 38
cellulite · 102, 104
    cedar essential oil · 38
    geranium essential oil · 38
    orange essential oil · 39
Celtic sea salt · 41, 139, 158
chamomile · 20, 23, 65, 70, 71, 73, 137, 145, 161
chamomile essential oil · 68, 70, 79, 96, 129, 161, 167

chamomile hydrosol · 65, 161
chaparral · 73
chickweed · 20, 21, 65, 70, 71, 73
children and babies · 36, 38, 139, 145
    chamomile · 23
    lavender · 24
chlorella · 158, 159
chlorophyll · 33, 65, 68, 71
Cinnamomum verum · 38
cinnamon · 20, 21, 61, 68, 130
cinnamon essential oil · 38, 61, 81, 83, 105, 130, 164
cistus essential oil · 71
citric acid · 54, 61, 77, 112, 113, 120, 149, 150
citrus · 39, 56, 61, 103, 134
Citrus sinensis · 39
clary sage essential oil · 68, 71, 139
clary sage hydrosol · 70, 71
cleavers · 21, 70
clove · 21, 130
clove essential oil · 61, 81, 169
cocoa butter · 33, 49, 65, 70, 71, 80, 82, 87, 88, 132, 143, 144
coconut oil · 49, 58, 65, 70, 71, 80, 82, 84, 85, 86, 87, 88, 90, 91, 93, 94, 95, 96, 112, 113, 120, 121, 132, 149, 150
Cocos nucifera · 49
colds · 85, 136, 147
    eucalyptus essential oil · 38
    ginger · 24
    mustard · 25
    orange essential oil · 39
    rosemary essential oil · 40
    tea tree essential oil · 40
colic · 145
comfrey · 20, 21, 23, 65, 70, 71, 73, 79
compress · 19
    plantain · 25
Copernicia cerifera · 49, 53
cornstarch · 53, 107
Corylus avellana · 45
cranberry · 34, 61, 65, 68, 70, 71
crystallization · *See* graininess
cumin essential oil · 61
cupuacu butter · 50, 65, 70, 71
Curcuma longa · 34
cuticles · 79, 93
cuts · 21, 79
    aloe vera · 22
    comfrey · 23
Cyampopis tetragonolobus · 53
cypress essential oil · 68, 86, 100

D

d-alpha tocopherol · *See* vitamin E
damiana · 156
dandruff · 22, 161, 167, 168, 169
    birch essential oil · 37
    cedar essential oil · 38
    cranberry · 34
    jojoba · 45
    sesame oil · 46
    tea tree essential oil · 40
dark hair · 161
dark spots · 114, 116
    apple cider vinegar · 55
    milk · 57
    rosehip seed oil · 46
    turmeric · 34
    yogurt. · 59
DEA · 18
Dead Sea salts · 42
deodorant · 89
    arrowroot · 52
    baking soda · 56
    chlorophyll · 34
    kaolin clay · 30
    sage · 27
detox · 148
diaper rash · 79, 89
    calendula · 22
diethanolamine · *See* DEA
digestive system · 66
distilled water · 120
dl-alpha tocopherol · *See* vitamin E
DMDM hydantoin · 18
dry brushing · 9
dry or sensitive skin chart · 70
dry plant oil · 74
dry shampoo · 29, 30, 57
dry skin · 117, 119, 122, 128, 143
    aloe vera · 22
    cocoa butter · 49
    jojoba · 45
    mango butter · 50
    sea buckthorn oil · 46
    sesame oil · 46
    shea butter · 51
dyes · 18

E

echinacea · 20, 73, 74, 79, 83
eczema · 20, 95, 119, 143
    almond oil · 44
    avocado oil · 45
    cupuacu oil · 50
    comfrey · 23
    geranium essential oil · 38
    kelp · 24
    kokum butter · 50
    lavender · 24
    neem · 45
    oats · 57
    plantain · 25
    rosehip seed oil · 46
    sea buckthorn oil · 46
    sesame oil · 46
    vegetable glycerin · 58
elder flower · 65, 68, 70, 71
emollient
    arrowroot · 52
    cupuacu oil · 50
    carnauba wax · 49, 53
    comfrey · 23
    kokum butter · 50
    rose essential oil · 39
emollient herbs · 20
epidermis · 65
Epsom salt · 42, 147, 148, 152, 154, 156
essential oil · 12, 18, 36, 45, 55, 57, 61, 66, 75, 76, 77, 79, 82, 84, 86, 88, 91, 94, 103, 112, 113, 119, 121, 132, 133, 134, 135, 136, 137, 142, 143, 144, 145, 148, 149, 150, 159, 161, 162, 165, 166
ethyl alcohol · 109, 110, 169
Eucaluptus radiata essential oil · 85
eucalyptus essential oil · 38, 39, 61, 68, 122, 147, 152, 169
Eucalyptus radiata · 38
evening primrose oil · 70, 71, 95, 96, 120
Everclear · *See* ethyl alcohol
exfoliate · 89, 105, 111, 126
    apple cider vinegar · 55
    milk · 57
    oats · 57
    sugar · 57
eye wash
    rose · 26
    self-heal · 27

F

facemask · 111
   bentonite clay · 29
   Fuller's earth · 30
   green clay · 30
   honey · 56
   kaolin clay · 30
   milk · 57
face toner · 117
   apple cider vinegar · 55
fatty acids · 45, 50, 54, 160
   kokum butter · 50
   rosehip seed oil · 46
   sea buckthorn oil · 46
   shea butter · 51
   walnut oil · 47
FD & C color pigments · 18
feet · 50, 87, 89, 100, 101, 106, 152, 153
   sage · 27
fennel · 65, 71
fennel essential oil · 71
fenugreek · 20, 70, 71
fever · 124
   self-heal · 27
fir essential oil · 143, 158
first aid · 83
   lavender essential oil · 38
   tea tree essential oil · 40
fixed oils · 25, 44, 49, 50, 53, 60, 61, 62, 109, 112, 119, 127, 133, 135, 159
flu · 40, 136, 147
   eucalyptus essential oil · 38
   ginger · 24
   orange essential oil · 39
   tea tree essential oil · 40
formaldehyde · 18
frankincense essential oil · 71
frankincense hydrosol · 68
free radicals
   annatto · 33
   cacao · 33
   cinnamon essential oil · 38
   rosemary · 27
   vitamin C · 59
fresh plant oil · 75
fruits and vegetables · 56
Fuller's earth · 30, 68
fungal infections · 152
fungus
   baking soda · 56
   yogurt · 59

G

Garcinia indica · 50
gargle
   comfrey · 23
   sage · 27
   self-heal · 27
garlic · 20, 21, 73
genetically modified · 53, 54
geranium · 20, 21, 68
geranium essential oil · 38, 65, 68, 70, 71, 88, 96, 100, 120, 127, 141
geranium hydrosol · 70, 71
German chamomile hydrosol · 70
ghassoul · *See* red clay
ginger · 21, 24, 98, 152, 158, 159
ginger essential oil · 81, 106
glycerol · *See* vegetable glycerin
goldenseal · 20
gotu kola · 71
graininess · 48, 84, 86
grape seed oil · 45, 68
grapefruit essential oil · 158
green clay · 30, 70, 71
green tea · 51, 61, 65, 70, 71
guar gum · 53
gum arabic · *See* acacia gum

H

hair · 56, 110, 160, 161, 162, 163, 165, 166, 167, 169, 170
   almond oil · 44
   apple cider vinegar · 55
   baking soda · 56
   cupuacu oil · 50
   clays · 29
   coconut oil · 49
   cranberry · 34
   guar gum · 53
   orange essential oil · 39
   rosemary · 26
   shea butter · 51
hair growth · 167
hair loss · 160
   rosemary essential oil · 40
Hawaiian red salt · 42
hazelnut oil · 45, 68, 70, 71

headache
    ginger · 24
    lavender · 24
    lavender essential oil · 38
    marjoram essential oil · 39
    peppermint essential oil · 39
helichrysum essential oil · 70, 71
helichrysum hydrosol · 70, 71
hemorrhoids · 97
    aloe vera · 22
    calendula · 22
    comfrey · 23
    self-heal · 27
hemostat
    comfrey · 23
    plantain · 26
    self-heal · 27
hemostat herbs · 21
herbal oils · 80, 82
herpes · 97
Himalayan salt · 42
Hippophae rhamnoides · 46
honey · 36, 56, 65, 68, 70, 71, 128
horsetail · 70, 161
hot flash · 124
humectant
    honey · 56
    sugar · 57
    vegetable glycerin · 58
hydrating · 57, 87, 117, 141
    rosehip seed oil · 46
    xanthan gum · 54
hydration · 143
hydrosol · 57, 112, 113, 150, 161

I

imidazolidinyl urea · 18
impurities · 102, 103
    bentonite clay · 29
    clays · 29
    Epsom salt · 42
infections · 85, 97, 119, 152
    baking soda · 56
    calendula · 22
    comfrey · 23
    lavender essential oil · 38
    marjoram essential oil · 39
    neem · 45
    peppermint essential oil · 39
    rose · 26
    rosemary essential oil · 40
    sage · 27
    tea tree essential oil · 40
infertility · 97
inflammation · 19, 20, 21, 44, 66, 95
    aloe vera · 22
    cranberry · 34
    kokum butter · 50
    lavender essential oil · 38
    sage · 27
    sea buckthorn oil · 46
injuries · 81
    calendula · 22
    lavender essential oil · 38
    rose · 26
insecticidal head lice treatments · 163
insects · 109
irritations · 79
    aloe vera · 22
    calendula · 22
    kelp · 24
    milk · 57
    oats · 57
    sage · 27
isopropyl alcohol · 18
itchy skin · 18, 95, 168
    cornstarch · 53
    lavender · 24
    rosehip seed oil · 46

J

jasmine essential oil · 65, 70, 71
jojoba · 45, 65, 68, 70, 71, 90, 93, 94, 100, 105, 120, 128, 134, 166, 169, 170
Juglans spp. · 47
juniper essential oil · 68, 102, 104, 154

K

kaolin clay · 30, 65, 68, 70, 71, 102, 103, 107, 126
karite butter · *See* shea butter
Kasturi turmeric · *See* turmeric
kelp · 24, 70, 71
keratin · 160
kidneys · 66
kokum butter · 50, 65, 68, 70, 71, 84, 86, 95, 96

L

lactic acid · 59
Laminaria spp. · 24
lanolin · 30, 80, 82, 112, 113, 120, 121
L-ascorbic acid · *See* vitamin C
Lavandula spp. · 24, 38
lavender · 24, 61, 65, 68, 70, 71, 73, 79, 89, 126, 137, 144, 145, 149, 156
   hydrosol · 57
lavender essential oil · 38, 39, 61, 65, 68, 70, 71, 88, 89, 91, 96, 107, 109, 120, 122, 127, 139, 117, 132, 134, 137
lavender hydrosol · 65, 68, 70, 71, 117, 120, 127
lead · 18
lecithin · 54
lemon · 102, 103
lemon balm · 25
lemon balm hydrosol · 68
lemon essential oil · 61, 68, 85, 89, 100, 102, 104, 109
lemon Eucalyptus essential oil · 68
lemon juice · 54, 68, 102, 169
lemon verbena hydrosol · 68
lemongrass essential oil · 68, 88, 89, 109, 124
licorice · 20, 68, 70, 98
lime juice · 169
lip balm · 32, 49, 80, 132, 134
liver · 24, 66
lymph · 66, 97, 102, 103, 105, 126, 155
   orange essential oil · 39

M

macadamia nut oil · 70, 71
magnesium · 30, 31, 33, 42, 43, 130
   kelp · 24
Mangifera indica · 50
mango butter · 50, 65, 70, 71, 93
Manihot esculenta · 58
Maranta arundinacea · 52
marjoram essential oil · 39, 137, 139, 154
marshmallow · 21, 70
Matricaria recutita · 23
mature skin · 71
   avocado oil · 45
   hydrosols · 57

mango butter · 50
rose essential oil · 40
rosehip seed oil · 46
sea buckthorn oil · 46
walnut oil · 47
mature skin chart · 71
MEA · 18
meadowsweet · 20
measurement conversions · 15
Melaleuca alternifolia · 40
Melissa · *See* lemon balm essential oil
Melissa officinalis · 25
memory
   rosemary · 26
Mentha piperita · 39
mica · 107, 132, 133, 134, 135
microbes · 61
milk · 57, 65, 68, 70, 71
mineral oxides · 34
moisturize · 44, 95
mold · 19, 60, 61, 63, 73, 75, 119
   citric acid · 61
molds · 88, 144, 150
momoethnanolamine · *See* MEA
Moroccan clay · *See* red clay
mrytle hydrosol · 70
mullein · 70, 73
muscle spasm
   rosemary · 26
mustard · 21, 147, 148
myrrh · 20, 130
myrrh essential oil · 70, 71

N

nails · 160
natural colorants · 149
neem · 45, 68, 120, 167
neroli essential oil · 65, 70, 71
nettles · 21, 161
normal skin chart · 65
nutmeg essential oil · 164
nutrients for the skin · 9

O

oak · 20, 21
oats · 57, 65, 68, 70, 102, 103, 126, 137, 156
oily and problem skin chart · 68

oily skin
    cedar essential oil · 38
    cranberry · 34
    Fuller's earth · 30
    grape seed oil · 45
    orange essential oil · 39
    red clay · 31
    tea tree essential oil · 40
Olea europaea · 46
olive oil · 44, 46, 65, 70, 71, 74, 95, 96, 120, 121, 164, 165
orange · 102
    hydrosol · 57
orange essential oil · 39, 68, 93, 102, 104, 106, 143, 158
orange flower · *See* neroli
orange flower hydrosol · 68, 69, 70, 71
oregano · 61, 68
oregano essential oil · 83, 164
Oregon grape · 20, 73
Origanum marjorana · 39
oxidation · 60

P

pain · 21, 81
    birch essential oil · 37
    cinnamon essential oil · 38
    cranberry · 34
    eucalyptus essential oil · 38
    kelp · 24
    lavender essential oil · 38
    mustard · 25
    peppermint essential oil · 39
    rosemary · 26
palmarosa essential oil · 68, 70, 71, 96
papaya · 56, 128
parabens · 18
patchouli essential oil · 70, 71
peach · 128
pear · 128
Pelargonium gravolens · 38
peppermint essential oil · 39, 85, 89, 100, 107, 109, 124, 130, 132, 134, 147, 152, 154, 161, 164, 169
peppermint hydrosol · 124
petrochemicals · 18
petroleum · 62
pH strip · 53, 114
phthalates · 18
pine essential oil · 85
Plantago major · 25

plantain · 20, 21, 25, 65, 70, 71, 73, 79
plastic pipettes · 133, 135
polyethylene glycol · 18
polysaccharides · 22, 52
pomegranate · 65, 70
poplar · 20, 21, 81
potassium sorbate · 61
preservatives · 18
problem skin · 117
    avocado oil · 45
    cranberry · 34
    eucalyptus essential oil · 38
propylene glycol · 18
Prunella vulgaris · 27
Prunus dulcis · 44
psoriasis
    almond oil · 44
    aloe vera · 22
    avocado oil · 45
    birch essential oil · 37
    comfrey · 23
    cranberry · 34
    plantain · 25
    sesame oil · 46
pyrrolizidine alkaloids · 24, 32

R

rancid oils · 44
rashes · 18
    aloe vera · 22
    calendula · 22
    green clay · 30
    kokum butter · 50
    lavender · 24
    oats · 57
    plantain · 25
    vegetable glycerin · 58
raspberry · 20
red clay · 31, 68
relaxing · 106, 139, 140, 156
    cedar essential oil · 38
    chamomile · 23
    lavender · 24
    lavender essential oil · 38
    marjoram essential oil · 39
rhassoul · *See* red clay
romantic · 141, 156
rooibos · 65, 68, 71
Rosa spp. · 26, 46

rose · 20, 26, 65, 68, 70, 71, 107, 137, 149, 156
    hydrosol · 57
rose essential oil · 39, 61, 65, 70, 71, 141
rose geranium · *See* geranium essential oil
rose hips · 61, 65, 71
rose hydrosol · 65, 68, 70, 71, 127, 141, 142, 149
rosehip seed oil · 46, 68, 70, 71, 112, 120
rosemary · 20, 21, 26, 61, 65, 68, 149, 161
    hydrosol · 57
rosemary antioxidant · 61, 95, 120
rosemary essential oil · 40, 61, 65, 68, 71, 88, 132, 134, 147, 154, 161, 167
rosemary hydrosol · 65, 68, 71, 161
rosewood essential oil · 156
rosmarinic acid · 40, 62
Rosmarinus officinalis · 26, 40
rubefacient
    mustard · 25
rubefacient herbs · 21

S

Saccharum officinarum · 57
sage · 20, 27, 61, 68, 73, 147, 148
sage essential oil · 61, 68, 137
Salvia officinalis · 27
sandalwood essential oil · 61, 68, 70, 71
scalp · 111, 160, 161, 162, 165, 166, 167, 168, 169, 170
    almond oil · 44
    cranberry · 34
scrapes · 21, 79
    lavender essential oil · 38
sea buckthorn oil · 46, 68, 70, 71, 112
sea salt · 41, 42, 130, 137, 156, 159
seborrheic dermatitis · *See* dandruff
sebum · 45
self-heal · 20, 27, 65, 68, 71, 73, 79
sensitive skin · 18, 114
    avocado oil · 45
    citric acid · 61
    green clay · 30
sesame oil · 46, 70
Sesamum indicum · 46
shea butter · 51, 65, 68, 70, 71, 84, 85, 86, 90, 91, 93

Simmondsia chinensis · 45
sitz bath · 97, 98, 99
    calendula · 22
    comfrey · 23
skin barrier · 48, 65, 93
skin care ingredients · 7, 18
skin elasticity
    hazelnut oil · 45
skin health · 8
skin types · 64
skin ulcers
    calendula · 22
    sea buckthorn oil · 46
sleep · 72, 139, 145
    chamomile · 23
    lavender · 24
    lemon balm · 25
sodium laureth sulfate · 18
sodium lauryl sulfate · 18
soothing · 20, 102, 137
    alkanet · 32
    aloe vera · 22
    calendula · 22
    comfrey · 23
    grape seed oil · 45
    kelp · 24
    lavender · 24
    lavender essential oil · 38
    lemon balm · 25
    oats · 57
    plantain · 25
sore muscles · 136, 155
    birch essential oil · 37
    cedar essential oil · 38
    Epsom salt · 42
    lavender · 24
    marjoram essential oil · 39
    rosemary essential oil · 40
    sage · 27
soy allergy · 54
spearmint essential oil · 130, 132, 134
spider bites
    bentonite clay · 29
spikenard essential oil · 70, 71
St. John's wort · 73, 75, 81
stearic acid · 50, 54, 112
stevia · 130
stimulating · 100, 158
    aloe vera · 22
    ginger · 24
    lavender essential oil · 38, 39
    mustard · 25
    peppermint essential oil · 39

stimulating *(cont.)*
　rosemary · 26
　rosemary essential oil · 40
stings · 79
　bentonite clay · 29
　lavender essential oil · 38
　plantain · 26
strawberries · 56
stress · 160
　lemon balm · 25
　orange essential oil · 39
　rose · 26
　sesame oil · 46
stretch marks
　aloe vera · 22
　calendula · 22
　cocoa butter · 49
　geranium essential oil · 38
　turmeric · 34
substitute for beeswax
　carnauba wax · 49, 53
substitute for cornstarch
　arrowroot · 52
　tapioca starch · 58
sugar · 57
sunburn
　aloe vera · 22
　apple cider vinegar · 55
　baking soda · 56
　kelp · 24
　lavender · 24
　oats · 57
　plantain · 25
　sea buckthorn oil · 46
　tea tree essential oil · 40
sunscreen · 89
sweating · 136
　calendula · 22
　ginger · 24
　mustard · 25
　sage · 27
Symphytum spp. · 23
synthetic colorants · 32
synthetic fragrances · 18, 36, 169
synthetic preservatives · 63

T

table salt · 26, 28, 41
talc · 107
tannins · 20
tapioca starch · 58

TEA · 18
tea tree essential oil · 40, 68, 83, 89, 107, 112, 117, 122, 152, 161, 164, 167
tempering butters · 48, 50, 51, 94, 96
Theobroma cacao · 33, 49
Theobroma grandiflorum · 50
thyme · 20, 61, 68
thyme essential oil · 61, 68, 83, 89, 109, 164
thyme linalool essential oil · 65, 85
titanium dioxide · 89
toluene · 18
toothpaste · 130
　baking soda · 56
　cinnamon essential oil · 38
　peppermint essential oil · 39
　tea tree essential oil · 40
travel · 87
triethanolamine · *See* TEA
turmeric · 20, 34, 68

U

uva ursi · 20, 98

V

Vaccinium spp. · 34
varicose veins · 101
　comfrey · 23
　rosemary essential oil · 40
　self-heal · 27
vegetable glycerin · 58, 65, 70, 71, 115, 116, 117, 122
vetiver essential oil · 70
vinegar · 36, 56
violet · 21, 65, 70, 71
vitamin C · 58, 65, 68, 70, 71, 112, 114, 116, 160
　beet · 33
vitamin E · 44, 46, 59, 62, 75, 76, 83, 85, 88, 90, 93, 95, 96, 105, 112, 120, 121, 132, 133, 134, 135, 159, 166
Vitellaria paradoxa · 51
Vitis vinifera · 45
vodka · 109, 110, 164, 165

vulnerary · 21
   calendula · 22
   plantain · 26
   slef heal · 27
vulnerary herbs · 21

W

walnut oil · 47, 65, 68, 71
whipped body butter · 51
willow · 20, 154
wintergreen · 21
witch hazel · 20, 21, 61, 65, 68, 71, 73,
   98, 100, 109, 110, 117, 122, 149, 150
   hydrosol · 57
witch hazel hydrosol · 65, 68, 71
wounds · 21, 97
   aloe vera · 22
   calendula · 22
   comfrey · 23
   Hawaiian red salt · 42
   mango butter · 50
   plantain · 26
   rose · 26
   sea buckthorn oil · 46

X

xanthan gum · 54, 70, 112
Xanthomonas camestris · 54
xylitol · 130

Y

yarrow · 20, 21, 65, 68, 73, 98, 100
yarrow essential oil · 70
yarrow hydrosol · 68, 71
yeast · 61
   tea tree essential oil · 40
ylang-ylang essential oil · 70, 137, 156
yogurt · 36, 59, 65, 66, 68, 70, 71, 102,
   103, 127, 128
yucca · 20

Z

Zea mays · 53
zinc oxide · 89
Zingiber officinale · 24

Recommended Resources

Most of the listed ingredients are readily available at your local herb or natural food store. If you can't find local sources, here are some high quality on-line resources that I have found to be reliable. I have also included places to find more information about the safety of skin care ingredients and household chemicals. I hope these recipes have inspired you. Please get creative, experiment, and have fun!

Supplies:

Mountain Rose Herbs
PO Box 50220
Eugene, OR 97405
(800) 879-3337
www.mountainroseherbs.com

Starwest Botanicals
161 Main Ave.
Sacramento, CA 95838
(800) 800-4372
www.starwest-botanicals.com

Frontier Herbs
3021 78th St.
Norway, IA 52318
(800) 669-3275
www.frontiercoop.com

Meadowsweet Herbs
180 South 3rd St West
Missoula, MT 59801
(406) 728-0543
www.meadowsweet-herbs.com

Sunburst Bottle
4200 Commerce Court Suite 206
Lisle, IL 60532
(877) 925-4500
www.sunburstbottle.com

New Directions Aromatics
840 Aero Drive - Suite 200
Cheektowaga, NY 14225
(800) 246-7817
www.newdirectionsaromatics.com

Samara Botane
P. O. Box 2483
Snohomish, WA 98291-2483
(800) 782-4532
www.wingedseed.com

From Nature With Love
341 Christian Street
Oxford, CT 06478
(800) 520-2060
www.fromnaturewithlove.com

Arlys
2033 W. McNab Road, Suite O
Pompano Beach, FL. 33069
(877) 502-7597
www.arlysnaturals.com

Herbal Information:

Green Path Herb School
P.O. Box 7813
Missoula MT 59807
(406) 274-2009
greenpathherbschool.com

United Plant Savers
PO Box 776
Athens, OH 45701
(740) 742-3455
 www.unitedplantsavers.org

American Botanical Council
6200 Manor Rd
Austin, TX 78723
(512) 926-4900
abc.herbalgram.org

American Herbalist Guild
125 South Lexington Ave. Suite 101
Asheville, NC 28801
(617) 520-4372
www.americanherbalistsguild.com

Jeanne Rose Institute of Aromatherapy & Herbal Studies
219 Carl St.
San Francisco, CA. 94117
415-564-6785
www.JeanneRose.net/courses.html

Information on Skin Care Products and Household Chemicals:

Women's Voices for the Earth
PO Box 8743
Missoula, MT 59807
(406) 543-3747
www.womensvoices.org

Skin Deep on-line Database
Environmental Working Group
1436 U St. NW #100
Washington DC 20009
www.ewg.org/skindeep/

A Consumer's Dictionary of Cosmetic Ingredients: Complete Information About the Harmful and Desirable Ingredients Found in Cosmetics and Cosmeceuticals by Ruth Winter

Milady's Skin Care and Cosmetic Ingredients Dictionary
by Natalia Michalun

Meves A, Stock SN, Beyerle A, Pittelkow MR, Peus D. Vitamin C derivative ascorbyl palmitate promotes ultraviolet-B-induced lipid peroxidation and cytotoxicity in keratinocytes. J Invest Dermatol 2002;119:1103-1108. (PubMed)

Herbs, Seeds and Plants:

Zach Woods Farm
278 Mead Rd
Hyde Park, VT 05655
(802) 888-7278
www.zackwoodsherbs.com

MoonBranch Botanicals
5294 Yellow Creek Road
Robbinsville, North Carolina 28771
(828) 479-2788
www.moonbranch.com

Friends of the Trees Society
PO Box 165
Hot Springs, MT 59845
(406) 741-5809
www.friendsofthetrees.net

Horizon Herbs
PO Box 69
Williams, OR 97544
(541) 846-6704
www.horizonherbs.com

Learn More About Herbs

Imagine you are walking through the forest near your home. As you look around, you start noticing the plants growing nearby. Imagine knowing each of these plants, understanding how to use them, when to harvest them and which parts to use. Envision being able to make these plants into medicines such as salves, oils, pills, syrups and tinctures. How would it feel to help others use these herbal medicines for healing purposes?

These are the skills of an herbalist. Are you ready to follow the path less traveled? Are you interested in deepening your connection with plants and the earth? Join us on a journey of exploration of medicinal herbs and natural remedies! We offer classes online and in person.

Our Offerings Include:
Free herbal information and recipes, natural health retreats, guest speaker workshops, on-line classes, wild-crafting trips, herb certificate programs and a school for training professional herbalists.

Find Out More:
Website: www.GreenPathHerbSchool.com
YouTube: http://www.youtube.com/user/greenpathherbschool
Facebook: https://www.facebook.com/Green.Path.Herb.School
Pinterest: http://pinterest.com/greenpathherb/boards/

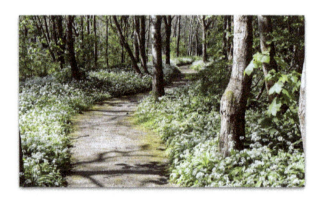

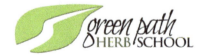

About the Author

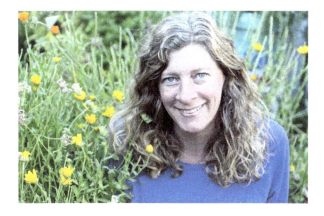

Elaine Sheff has been studying medicinal plants since 1987. A Clinical Herbalist, she is a graduate of both the Rocky Mountain Center for Botanical Studies and the Southwest School of Botanical Medicine. Elaine is a certified instructor of Fertility Awareness and Natural Family Planning, a safe, effective natural birth control method used to avoid or achieve pregnancy. She has a long-standing clinical practice providing herbal consultations for individuals with health concerns. A best selling author, Elaine teaches herb classes throughout the United States. She was the co-founder of Meadowsweet Herbs and is the co-director of Green Path Herb School in Missoula, Montana. You can often find Elaine in her garden, spending time with her amazing family, or cooking gluten free.

Other Books by Elaine Sheff:

Natural Remedies for the Fall: Preparing for Cold & Flu Season

Herbal Love Potions: Natural Recipes to Celebrate Romance and Sensuality

CPSIA information can be obtained
at www.ICGtesting.com
Printed in the USA
BVHW091104170719
553682BV00017B/1185/P